FINE, THANKS

Stories from the Cancerland Jungle

Mary Dunnewold

Black Rose Writing | Texas

The author grants the final approval for this literary material.

Second printing

Some names and identifying details may have been changed to protect the privacy of individuals.

ISBN: 978-1-68433-378-3
PUBLISHED BY BLACK ROSE WRITING
www.blackrosewriting.com

Printed in the United States of America
Suggested Retail Price (SRP) $18.95

Fine, Thanks is printed in Palatino Linotype

To Jeff

Acknowledgements

I owe a huge debt of gratitude to the many, many people who supported me during my cancer treatment and who continue to make my life rich and full, no matter what comes my way. First, thank you to all the wonderful doctors, nurses, and other medical practitioners who cared for me during this time. I don't know all of your names, but every one of you contributed to my survival. Special thanks to my legion of friends in Northfield and elsewhere for the gifts, food, words of encouragement, and time spent shoring me up, especially to Carolyn Link, Rob Hardy, Clara Hardy, Jackie Rolfs, David Severtson, Susan Sanderson, Anne Meyer-Ruppel, Mary Carlson, Jane Blockhus, Sarah Bardenwarper, Mary Carlsen, Mary Upham, Kathryn Jamison, Anne Larson, Sarah Currier, Patrice O'Morchoe, Carolyn Chalmers, and Eric Janus. My colleagues at Hamline University School of Law, especially Mary Trevor, Beth Honetschlager, Ken Swift, and Brenda Tofte, made it possible for me to continue to teach and thrive professionally during this difficult chapter. Thank you to Amy and all the wonderful teachers at Heartwork Yoga Studio for the encouragement and free yoga. Thank you to my sisters, Jane, Ann, and Ruth, my mother Elinor, the Ondich clan, and all of my extended family, for being the best ever. And, of course, to Elena, Sam, and Jeff for making it all worthwhile.

FINE, THANKS

Chapter One

In the six months before I had cancer, I fell down three times.

First, in January, on a barely frozen Saturday morning, a silvering of ice on every surface. But the dog had to be walked. The dog, bred for pulling freight in the northern wilds. It was not her fault. She threatened to topple me on the driest of surfaces, in mid-July, when my flip-flops adhered to the sun-melted asphalt. But now, in the ice-shrouded January, she was standing still. I moved the tiniest bit, just to make way for the neighbor's car, careening around the corner. The unfriendly neighbor, out to buy grocery-store donuts on Saturday morning.

Was it careening? I can't remember. Anything that moved that morning was careening, because of the ice-bound stillness, the rigidity of the trees.

I stood still, but then stepped aside, the tiniest step, to avoid the careening car, watching where I put my foot down.

Not a dry patch. I thought it was a dry patch. But it was hard to tell, on that ice-glittery morning. Nothing was dry. Nothing was to be trusted.

I went down, not even like a cartoon character, not even flailing my arms and legs. I went down at the command of gravity and friction, or anti-friction, just down. My arm cracked, just like that. Crack, and it's broken, obviously.

What do you do, then, when you go down, and your arm has cracked, and the dog is sniffing your face with her big watery nose, wondering: What new game is this? While you gaze up, stunned, at the indifferent, prison-grey sky? And your neighbor, unfriendly despite the cookies you took to his sullen wife and unruly children, at least stops to say, are you all right? And you say, I think I broke my arm. And he says, oh. Then gets back into his car, and pulls into his snout-house garage, which is tacked onto an exact specimen of the uncharming, beige houses of the suburbs. And the garage door shuts quietly behind him, because of the silent, inexplicable physics of the ice world.

Strike one.

The second time was in public. I never wear heels. I wore heels. The "new" me. Look at me, I can wear heels. A last-ditch attempt at sexy youth, having spent my actual sexy youth wearing only comfy shoes, canvas and plastic, which I sometimes decorated with Crayola markers. Sexy Shoes as the Great Experiment of the Aging Feminist.

I was wearing a dress, even, and nylons, and heels. The restaurant was trendy, but not that great. Not good enough for a dress, and nylons, and heels. But never mind. We were dressed up and on a date. I think my husband, Jeff, was even wearing a jacket, but who knows. He only owns one, and it pretty much stays put on the red plastic hanger in the back of the closet, nursing a chronic case of agoraphobia.

I'd only had one drink. Really. It was not the drink. It was the ice (again). This time, the tiniest piece of ice, not the great, unavoidable swath of ice. I was striding through the trendy, not-that-great restaurant, down the narrow gangplank between the bar and the tables, because the whole place was quite small, actually. Intimate.

Suddenly, more like a cartoon character this time, a cartoon character on a banana peel. Except there was no banana peel. I was down.

It was just a tiny piece of ice, mostly melted. I store the memory of it in my right foot, where it imprinted through the thin sole of my imposter dress-up shoes. I went down, just like that, my traitorous skirt flying up around my waist.

There was a gasp, and many diners half-rose out of their chairs, responding to the visceral call, the altruistic gene. Attention: Member of herd is down! A waiter ran over to help me up. My husband offered me his hand.

No, No. Fine. I'm fine. Really.

I'm not drunk, damn it.

Ice on the floor. I tell you.

Strike two.

The third time was my Near Death Experience. A casual fall on a mossy step, head missing the corner by an inch. I already had cancer at this point. At least my body had cancer. *I* did not yet have cancer because my brain did not yet know that my body had cancer. You can't *have* cancer until your body and your brain cooperate in this matter.

Anyway, I ask you: If there is A Plan for Me, forged by The Universe (about which I have grave doubts), why would I survive this near-death fall, with only a few-day's stiff neck as remembrance, just to be preserved for the ordeal of advanced-stage cancer, chemotherapy, radiation, eight surgeries, multiple infections, and a subclavian blood clot? Wouldn't it have been better to die quickly, in that hapless fall, in a moistly green, temperate paradise, on a morning hike with my sweetheart, because the wooden steps into the ravine were damp from a passing shower?

My answer to that question, even now, is: No. It would not have been better to die in a tragic fall, a few months before my cancer diagnosis, before I *had* cancer, and thus not actually live to *have* cancer.

I have wanted to live every minute since I was diagnosed with cancer.

•   •   •   •   •

There is a moment when you pass through the threshold, the gossamer curtain, the liminal ectoplasm, from not having cancer to having cancer. Like moving from "not-parent" to "parent." "Parent" did not happen the moment my first-born entered the physical world. Rather, it happened when, returning from the hospital on that sunny Tuesday in June, I reached towards the screen door, green paint peeling, the latch a little rusty around the edges, and thought: my life will never be the same. And when I entered the house, plastic car seat handle digging into my arm, the baby squirming in his bucket, life as I knew it was over.

With cancer, it was the mammogram technician's eyes. Or averting thereof. Her refusal to look up from my chart as she explained that she "just needed a sec" for the radiologist to take a look. Consigning me to Pink Gown Purgatory while she went out, for just a sec.

When she hurried back in, the radiologist bustling behind her, his eyes on my films, I knew I had passed through that curtain. The bustling, the hurry, had an exaggerated physical quality, as if it could fill the chasm yawning in front of me with movement and sound. Or at least provide a diversion. Like in the video of the selective attention experiment, where you never notice the guy in the gorilla suit, strolling through the basketball game, because you are so focused on the game itself. Me, the radiologist, and the mammogram tech, all suited up for basketball. Cancer in the gorilla suit.

I'd had a clear mammogram in January 2010, six months earlier. They'd called me back for "a few more views," then concluded I was fit for service for another year. But I'd been called back in other years, and biopsied in two of them. In fact, call-backs had become fairly routine. Like forgetting to write my name on math papers in fifth grade. Kind of troublesome, but no harm done in the end.

But in July that year, the last Monday in July, before the Thursday eye-avertings, there it was. A lump.

I had pretty much dispensed with self-exams. The latest research showed they didn't accomplish much, really. But my annual exam appointment was on Tuesday, so on Monday, in the shower, hmm, I wonder if they're right about that. I'd hate to go in and have a massive lump I never noticed. How irresponsible. How careless. Like driving with your blinker on *and* your gas cap hanging open.

My fingers went right to it, as if my body knew I had cancer and was done waiting for me to figure it out. Okay, brain, don't over-think this. Here's the lump.

Left side. About seven o'clock. Not that I usually think of my breasts as clocks.

It wasn't much of a lump, really. More like a weirdly grainy area. Not like the lump in the fake boob we passed around, some of us grimacing, some giggling, in ninth grade health class; plastic breast with ready-made cancer. (Where were the boys that day anyway? Feeling up fake testicles?)

But that tiny step through the gossamer curtain did not occur on that Monday in the shower, or even on Tuesday, when my doctor, looking thoughtful, prodded the area. Grainy, she pronounced. Let's do a mammogram.

Maybe I'm wrong, but I believe she looked at my name on her schedule as a bright spot in her day, not as a cancer candidate. I am what is known as "compliant." In fact, I am the queen of compliance. Exams, screenings, immunizations—I'm on board. I don't smoke or fool around. I drink some wine on the weekend, but that's good for my heart, right? I call ahead for prescription refills. I eat organic and do yoga. I wear my seatbelt and my bike helmet, and yes, I feel safe at home. My father, tragically, died too early of dementia, but otherwise my relatives die of old age, counting the days. My worst vices are expensive chocolate and Grey's Anatomy.

Besides, we liked to swap titles of recent good reads while she probed my nether regions.

So I made the mammogram appointment for Thursday morning. Despite the "grainy" pronouncement, I wasn't worried. I could wait until Thursday.

I went to work, met with colleagues, came home, and walked the dog, made dinner with friends. It was corn-on-the-cob season. There is nothing like an ear of corn harvested in the lush, verdant Minnesota fields a few hours earlier and sold from the back of the Larson family's red pickup by fresh-faced midwestern teenagers in the parking lot of Gina's Hair Palace. Boil until slightly tender, three to five minutes, and finish with a generous sprinkling of salt and a smear of pale yellow butter. On the list of things worth living for, corn-on-the-cob season in Minnesota is at the top. I ate lots.

Even Thursday morning, when I could not have better staged a real-life Stupid Metaphor, I wasn't really worried.

Stupid Metaphor Number One. I was fussing around in the kitchen, hurrying to clean up so I would make my 8:30 appointment at the clinic. I don't know how it happened. I swear I didn't touch it. No ice was involved.

My favorite drinking glass, the lone remnant of a four-glass set, a wedding present in 1984, shattered.

These were quality glasses. Not cheap Target junk that breaks into dagger-like shards that you pick up one by one and toss in the trash. It shattered into a thousand little crystalline pieces (okay, I know, literature has been here before, but this actually happened) and they went everywhere.

I thought: give me a freaking break. Off to get the cancer mammogram, and my favorite glass shatters as I go out the door. I can't possibly have cancer, because that would be the stupidest thing that has ever happened to me.

But, of course, I did have cancer. And I was only a few eye-avertings and a gorilla basketball game away from knowing it.

·　　·　　·　　·　　·

So a few hours later that Thursday morning, I was in a procedure room, bared to the waist, slathered with betadine, needle poised for the assault. My appointment had been for 8:30 a.m. I had spent a few minutes first in the stupidly pink waiting room, waiting for the mammogram tech to appear, paging through *Glamour* magazine. (Only in waiting rooms. I have principles.) It was now 8:50 a.m.

Those rooms are dimly lit, as if it's date night with the radiologist. I'm sure there is a perfectly good medical-scientific explanation. Screens, ultrasound images, the necessity of eye avertings. Or maybe not. Maybe it's about keeping the half-naked, shivering woman, who is envisioning her motherless children and her husband's remarriage to the cute divorcee down the block, from finding the door.

The voices were all so deliberately soothing. The radiologist was so nice. He apologized profusely with every *SNAP* of the biopsy extractor, which sounds something like a staple gun.

Okay hold really still, I'm going to count to three, then you'll hear a snap, okay? Ready? One. Two. Three. *SNAP*. Sorry. Really sorry about that. Okay hold really still again, I'm going to count to three, then you'll hear a snap, okay? Ready? One. Two. Three. *SNAP*. Sorry about that. Really sorry.

Okay, I get it. You're sorry. One two three *Snap*. Just do it and get me the hell out of here.

The blond women in pink scrubs had multiplied, the eye averters. There was one to open the plastic packaging on the equipment, one to guide the phallic ultrasound wand across the terrain of my left breast, and one to pat me on the shoulder and help me pretend I did not have cancer. I wondered if my husband would marry the divorcee or just go back and forth between houses at odd hours, out of respect for the children.

Your doctor will call you. Probably tomorrow afternoon. Leave your number with the nurse.

•   •   •   •   •

I got into my car and sped through those lush July cornfields, a little lead in my foot. I had a long work commute from my bucolic Minnesota small town to the law school where I taught in St. Paul, forty-five miles away. I'd been commuting for sixteen years, and I listened to audiobooks as I drove, because otherwise I would have put a gun to my head about five years earlier.

I plugged in my iPod and on came a book about a woman who has died of cancer haunting the apartment she shared with her husband.

Not a metaphor, like the shattering glass that morning, but really? I don't actually believe in The Universe Speaking to Me, but please.

I switched to public radio instead. Minimal chance of cancer there. Although you never know. I have since noticed that cancer pops up everywhere when you are least expecting it. I listened for a few minutes and decided it was safe.

I stopped in suburban Eagan, halfway to Saint Paul, to buy bagels. My son Sam, my first born, skinny child, has Crohn's Disease, and at the time, he didn't like to eat. Eating made his life miserable, pretty much. There were stretches where he lived on raspberry white chocolate chip scones from the local coffeehouse (can you put a few more calories into that scone, please?) and Homestyle Chicken Noodle Soup from a can. But he liked plain bagels, as long as they were fresh and had just the right amount of regular, not reduced fat, cream cheese.

I would do pretty much anything to get Sam to eat. And on that day, I could feel a crisis of the psyche coming on. I was about to lose my natural source of nourishment for my children, my breasts, while already carrying a boatload of guilt about being unable to feed my child. So I stopped for bagels.

As I pulled out of the bagel strip mall, across six lanes of suburban traffic, my car started protesting. THWUMP. THWUMP. THWUMP.

Stupid Metaphor Number Two.

I pulled into a strip mall parking lot and put the car in park. Got out and examined the tires. Thought they looked okay. Got back in. Pulled back into traffic.

THWUMP. THWUMP. THWUMP.

I made my way onto the highway overpass, conflicted about whether to turn left onto the northbound ramp and continue on to work or stop for further investigation.

THWUMP. THWUMP. THWUMP.

I pulled to the right and squeezed onto a tiny shoulder of pavement just after the overpass. Cars zoomed by. How odd that the world was oblivious to the fact that not only did I appear to have cancer, but now I also had a flat tire.

I sat there for a few minutes, on hold for the roadside service operator. My father raised four feminist daughters, but I have my limits.

A police car pulled in behind me, and the officer appeared at my window. You're not parked in a very safe spot, Ma'am. Can you pull around the corner?

7

No, I can't possibly pull around the corner. Not only do I have a flat tire, I have cancer.

Yes, of course. Sorry to cause trouble. You're sure it won't damage my wheel rim? Or make my cancer worse?

I have to say, maybe it's just Minnesota. (Don't move here. It's really cold, and we like the fact that it's not as crowded as the coasts.) But as I sat there for the next forty-five minutes, around the corner, waiting for the tow truck to rescue me, seven people stopped to ask, Need Help?

In fact, I do.

But don't worry. Help is on the way.

I sat in my car, July sun pulsing on the roof, but not unpleasant with the windows cranked wide, talking to my sister Ann, pausing periodically to tell a Fellow Minnesotan that, no thanks, I did not need help.

Then, after my tow-truck rescue, I turned around south and drove home, on my wobbly spare tire, where I left the car in the capable hands of the neighborhood mechanic, walked the few blocks to my house, went upstairs, and not for the last time in the next few weeks, climbed into bed and pulled the covers over my head.

•   •   •   •   •

Thursday evening, I looked at Jeff, my husband, as he shucked the corn-on-the-cob across the kitchen island from me. Jeff is my rock. He likes to note that he is a Taurus born in the year of the Bull. Double solid, but more like Ferdinand than Durham. He teaches computer science at the local college. During the summer, when he doesn't teach, he sits in his comfy chair in the living room, occasionally rising to navigate the golden triangle of chair, fridge, and bathroom, and writes computer code, doing his part to keep the world safe from inelegant software. I know he'll be there, in his chair, when I come home, and if he's not, he's out walking the dog.

I was trying not to worry Jeff, so I wasn't really talking to him about the cancer thing much. I hadn't told him about the lump on Monday. After the doctor's appointment on Tuesday, I told him I'd scheduled a mammogram, but I wasn't worried, it was pretty routine. After the mammogram on Thursday, I'd told him, yeah, they did a biopsy, but I think it will be fine. Why pull him into this anxiety pit a minute earlier than need be? He had better things to do than worry about me.

Fortunately, in my mind anyway, my daughter, Elena, was across town (okay, six blocks away because that's just the kind of town it is) in a residential science camp for several weeks, and Sam was twenty and had a scooter. What socially connected, charming twenty-year-old boy with a scooter spends any time at home with his parents in the heart of a beautiful Minnesota July, even if he does have Crohn's Disease? He mainly seemed to pop in for the occasional bathroom break and bagel. So I could let Jeff code away and mostly keep my thoughts to myself.

I'm not worried, I told myself. Don't worry, I told myself.

But of course, I was worried.

Would telling Jeff have made it more real? By externalizing my worry, would anything have changed? Telling someone might have meant admitting I needed help. And I was not very good at that at the time. Much as you might want to, you can't get through cancer without some help.

But I was new to cancer, and I had some learning to do.

· · · · ·

The next day, Friday, I did go to work.

But not at first. First, Jeff and I met with our adorable financial planners, Kit and Jeremy, at our dining room table. Jeremy reminds me of a Golden Retriever puppy. Perennially cute, blond, with wide, eager eyes. Bringing the ball of financial planning decisions back to your lap again and again, even when you're sick of thinking about it and would rather stick a knife in your eye. Kit is cute too, how can he not be with a name like Kit, but in a slightly more earnest way.

Here is another area where I (or rather, we, meaning the heroic Jeff and I) manage our life well. We save. We can cover college for the kids. We don't spend money we don't have. In almost three decades of marriage, we have not accrued a penny of interest on a credit card, except that time Jeff asked his friend Bruce to drop the bills in the mailbox and instead they got lost on the floor of Bruce's Honda for several months. Shouldn't this compliance buy you some Universal Approbation (meaning anti-cancer insurance) somewhere? Otherwise, why bother?

So we sat at the dining room table talking about the demise of social security, the rising cost of college, our "financial goals," and the merits of the TIAA CREF Social Choice Fund versus the TIAA CREF Equal

Justice Fund. Jeremy was a little down at the mouth because we hadn't told him quite far enough in advance that we were going to need a certain chunk of money for a certain forgettable purpose, and it probably cost us a few percentage points in interest for a couple of weeks, to the tune of about fifty bucks. In short, we'd been distracted and failed to throw the ball. Sorry Jeremy.

College. Retirement. Trips to Paris and Thailand. My daughter's wedding.

Would I be around for that stuff?

Because I hadn't told him much, I'm pretty sure Jeff did not realize just how surreal it was to sit through two hours of Planning for the Future when I already knew I had cancer, but I couldn't yet say so. I couldn't say to Kit and Jeremy: I will definitely be dead in six months, so you really should add an extra $250,000, the proceeds from my life insurance, into that total there. That should top off the college fund *and* pay for the wedding, given that Elena will not be an extravagant bride. (She was definitely on track to be a wedding-in-the-park, followed by a potluck, kind of bride.)

They left, with promises to meet again in a year for our annual financial check-up. Yeah, right. You three have fun.

Then I went to work. Because what else are you going to do while you wait?

• • • • •

It's a long afternoon when you are waiting for that call. You spend some time feeling sorry you're making the doctor's day harder. How awful, delivering terrible news on Friday afternoon. Does she put it off all day because she can't see another patient after that? Or is four o'clock really when the lab results arrive?

Then you realize that after the doctor delivers the news, she packs up her doctor tools, locks the clinic door, and goes home to a weekend of boating or poolside reading, or whatever she spends her doctor money on. Whereas you spend the weekend thinking about whether you're going to die.

You obsessively check your phone for messages, even though the ringer is turned on high and the vibrate is on, and the phone nestles in your pocket, right next to your body, so even if a truck rumbled through the room, you would still feel it tickling your thigh. Every few minutes, you take it out of your pocket and switch the ringer on and off, just to make sure, and check the battery level while you're at it.

I didn't want to take the call in the car because, being so compliant and all, I am a firm believer in not talking on the phone while driving. Besides, I'd been commuting two hours a day for twenty years. I was statistically much more likely to die in a fiery crash than to die of cancer. Combining the risk of the former with the emotional devastation of the latter did not seem like a good plan. But my doctor hadn't called by 3:30, and I had a haircut appointment with Samantha at Buzz in an hour. And if there is one thing you don't get in the way of, it's a haircut appointment with Samantha. So I got in the car and headed to Northfield.

I almost made it there. The phone rang just as I headed down the exit ramp from the interstate and got ready to turn east, down the green, corn-lined corridor that would take me into town. I flipped open the phone and told my doctor I was driving. She said, Well, why don't you pull over. I can wait.

Those are not the words you want to hear from your doctor. I can wait. Doctors don't Wait for You. You Wait for Them. That's one of the Rules of the Universe.

I pulled onto a tiny shoulder of road. The corn corridor was being rebuilt, and it was hot and noisy and reeked of asphalt. The asphalt rollers and front-end loaders rumbled around me like alien insects on steroids. There was nowhere else to park. If a police officer came to my window this time, I was going to hand him the phone. Let him take the hit.

It is a cancer, she said. We don't know much yet, but it's blah blah positive and blah blah other positive, which is the most common blah blah, but blah blah Monday when I'm not in, so blah blah blah. Okay?

Down. Crack.

Indifferent sky. Dog's nose. What new game is this?

.   .   .   .   .

It still seems odd that the first person I told was Samantha, my hair stylist. In retrospect, that seems disrespectful to my family and dearest friends, but also to Samantha. What was she supposed to do with that information? She was in no position to comfort me. To offer advice. To tell me everything would be okay.

But there I was, ten minutes later in Samantha's chair, with the black cape protecting me from the potential of itch. She asked me how I was. I said fine. Fine. We chatted about my kids, and whether my daughter would ever cut her freakishly long hair. About how Samantha's business was getting on in the beautiful heart of July, when there are no college kids around with money to spend on haircuts. About the vintage car rally scheduled on Main Street for that weekend. I made it all the way to the end of the appointment, but as she was dusting the remaining bits of hair off my neck with the soft whisk-like brush that reminds me of my father's old-fashioned shaving brush, I couldn't stop myself.

She asked if I wanted to schedule for six weeks out, as usual. I said: I was just diagnosed with breast cancer an hour ago. On my way home. I don't know if I'll have hair in six weeks.

She looked stricken. It was a perfectly innocent, business-like question, after all. She had not said, You're looking a touch peaked today. Maybe a little pale. Do you have cancer?

Poor Samantha.

•   •   •   •   •

You think you are taking care of yourself, running a good shop. The organic food. The yoga. The years of therapy and regular massages. Even the financial hygiene. You think: I am doing everything right. Master of my Universe.

When Sam was a senior in high school, he had a girlfriend named Maddy, a waif-like girl with very white skin, intensely red hair that seemed to remain in a "pixie" cut no matter how much time passed, and big brown eyes. She was vivacious and adorable. Definitively elfin.

Maddy's mother was French. Actual French, like from-France French. Maddy's grandparents lived in France, and she went to visit them over spring break that year. They took her shopping in Paris for her prom dress. This girl was definitely doing everything right. Equally adorable Sam, done up in his father's slim-cut wedding suit, had a tie that exactly matched Maddy's hair. He had purchased a wrist corsage for her rather than a pin-on since there was nowhere to pin anything on the bodice of her dress.

When they got to prom, another girl, a frumpy, un-cool girl (maybe I just imagined that part), came up to Maddy and asked her where she got her dress. The girl was wearing exactly the same dress. She'd gotten it at Macy's. Twenty miles up the highway at the Burnsville mall.

This story nudged me as I struggled to make sense of my diagnosis. The moral of the story fit my mood: No matter how compliant you are, no matter how much good fortune you enjoy, bad luck can strike at any time.

Don't think you're so special. Don't think you're exempt.

·   ·   ·   ·   ·

So far, I have survived cancer, as you can see. But I may never be sure what "surviving cancer" means. Is there a statute of limitations on cancer? I've passed the portentous five-year survival mark, but I only take so much comfort in that. How do I know it's not still lurking out there in some hepatic backwater, waiting for round two? Once you have stepped through the curtain, do you ever step back? Is that morning low back pain a mid-life bulging disk, traceable to that one extra shovelful of snow? Or is it cancer? These questions trouble me still, years later, even though I feel great. I may never move entirely out from under their shadow.

And my magical thinking, a belief that somehow, because I struck out once, I could strike out again, persisted. A few years ago, we were living for a while in an apartment in Minneapolis, a post-cancer experiment with changing up our life. I was trotting into the kitchen in my bathrobe and bare feet to get filtered water from the fridge door for my neti pot. (See? I even use a neti pot. Shouldn't I get credit for that?) It was Saturday, and I had spent an enjoyable morning puttering— straightening up, wiping down the fridge, watering the plants—while singing along to hits from the Eighties. I was getting ready to move on to the "home spa" hour: self-facial, nail trimming, errant hair removal, long hot shower with an expensive body scrub.

A few minutes earlier, I had traversed the same path with the dripping watering can. The floor was shiny, new, not-quite wood, and a little wet. And it was slipperier than I realized.

Down. Crack.

Game two, strike one?

Chapter Two

For a while, the dismay at finding yourself in this predicament—are you a cancer "survivor" before you even begin treatment?—and your pointless puzzlement over what got you here, with no apparent warning, is overcome by the practical realities pressing on your daily life. The immediate problem is: how do you tell people?

At first, I thought: maybe I won't tell anyone. I look perfectly healthy. I feel perfectly fine. I could do nothing for a long time, and no one would know. There are some things you only tell your hair stylist, right?

Besides, at first, I was sure it was only a tiny bit of cancer. Just a wee mite of a cancer. Surely I would go in next week, they would nip out a little piece, and then stitch me up, good as new. But I would need to sob for a few hours, for which I would need a shoulder, or at least an explanation. And I'd need a ride.

So I decided I should at least tell Jeff.

When I pulled up to our house after my haircut that Friday afternoon, Jeff was across the street talking to our neighbor, Kathryn. Kathryn had planted a prairie in her front yard that year, and it was in full glorious bloom. In fact, the whole neighborhood was lush and beautiful. The yards were shaded by mature oaks and maples and bounded by abundant perennials, and the smell of fresh cut grass was always in the air. The sounds of children playing at the nearby community pool only enhanced the perfection of the summer day. Ours is the textbook small town, the classic setting for the American Dream. We often joked about living in a bubble, where it seemed that nothing could ever go wrong.

But of course, things went wrong. And now I was a reminder of that.

Jeff loves talking to Kathryn so he would not normally run right over home when I pull into the driveway. Rather, it would be up to me to go over and join them. But he had his cancer-seeking radar on, and he is, after all, a pretty sensitive guy who was waiting for my news that afternoon. So he said goodbye to Kathryn and caught up with me as I exited the garage.

I looked past his shoulder at the squirrels stealing seeds from the bird feeder. I should do something about those squirrels, I thought.

It's cancer, I said. Then I started to cry right there in the driveway.

Jeff put his arms around me and walked me into the house, where I sobbed out what I knew so far. We sat on the sofa, and he held me while I cried and fetched me water and tissues and told me it would be okay. But this initial storm didn't last that long. There was really nothing to do. I didn't have cancer, then I did. I didn't know much more than that.

So Jeff took out his phone and called the local Indian restaurant, which he has on speed dial, and ordered some food. He went to pick it up while I changed into my comfiest clothes and washed my face. When he returned, he got out the plates, loaded them up, and pushed me gently towards the sofa, where I ate my spicy Indian food, but barely tasted it, while we watched a movie. So, pretty much a normal Friday night. Because normal Friday nights make up your life, and your life keeps ticking away, minute by minute, no matter what obstacles fall in your path.

The next morning, I lay awake for a while, the early-rising summer sun streaming through the bedroom window, thinking about who to tell and what to tell them. Jumping in there too quickly risked establishing the wrong tone entirely. Guess what?! I have cancer! Couldn't wait to tell you!

But waiting too long seemed problematic too. By the way. Had my breasts removed last week. Didn't want to bother you, but thought you might like to know since it means I can't be at rehearsal tonight.

There had to be a sweet spot. A middle ground.

I climbed out of bed and headed to the bathroom to brush my teeth because the dog had to be walked before it got too warm. In the bathroom, I pulled off my sleep shirt and looked in the mirror. Now that my brain and body had cooperated and I knew without a doubt that I had cancer, it seemed amazing that the only visible signs of my predicament were the band-aids covering the biopsy punctures. Otherwise, I was as healthy as I'd been the previous Saturday, when I'd climbed out of bed in northern Minnesota, taken a moderately strenuous five-mile hike, and driven three hours home to the usual "I've got the end of vacation blues but let's get back to work" feeling. Shouldn't my life have changed since yesterday? When had I actually crossed from healthy to potentially doomed? When had that cell, then cluster of cells, gone rogue, sending my life careening off in this direction? Shouldn't I have been able to feel that moment happen?

I pulled a t-shirt over the field of band-aids on my chest, then went downstairs and harnessed up the dog, Ruby.

Ruby and I headed down the sidewalk under the shady trees, stopping here and there so she could sniff the doggy morning news. As we walked, I decided on a three-tiered communication strategy.

Tier One: my mother and immediate family. I would do that right after the walk. Phone calls. Probably some crying involved, but I would do my best to hold it together.

Tier Two: good friends—the kind that, if you run into them and they ask you how you are, you actually tell them. Couldn't risk losing it at the coffee shop, so it needed to be done soon. I planned to lay low that day and not run into anyone, so that could be Saturday evening, after I'd had time to think through the words, accomplished with one group email.

Tier Three: work authority figures and work friends. Sunday, by email. That way, no one would expect me to show up on Monday, but they wouldn't feel like they needed to do anything about it before then. Anyone who did not fall into one of these categories would hear it from someone else soon enough.

This put me in the position of categorizing the people who populate my life into a kind of rank order. I've always hated ranking games.

Top ten movies? Uh...conversation moves on before my brain communicates a plausible response to my mouth, even though this question comes up possibly once a month.

Top ten songs? Well, do you count just "songs," technically, or would you consider symphonic movements to be "songs"? How about tone poems? Operatic arias? Movie scores? Ringtones?

Top five moments in high school? Give me a break. There were no good moments in high school.

Also, the finer details of my plan were not quite clear yet. In what order should I call my sisters? Birth order? Affinity? Alphabetical? Should I include my children in Tier One, or are they a special sub-category, mavericks, because they still need me to protect them from the big scary world? Did my work friend Mary, who I sometimes saw outside of work, count in Tier Two or Tier Three?

I'd only "had" cancer for a few hours, and already my life was so complicated.

Ruby and I took an extra-long walk while I thought this all through, and then, back at home, I settled myself on the screen porch with my phone, a box of Kleenex, and a cup of tea.

First, I called my mother. After her cheerful hello, before she could launch into the usual topics—the weather, the church news, the litany of what was in bloom—I blurted it out. "I have breast cancer."

There was a terrible pause in which I wished I could take it back. My mother was almost eighty years old, and other than my Father's distressing descent into early dementia and its consequences, had lived a pretty tragedy-free life. Good genes. No cancer, heart disease, or diabetes—I came by it honestly. Besides, parents don't want to think they might outlive their children. That went out of style in the early twentieth century. How could I be doing this to her?

And she had always exhibited an insuppressible optimism. I would call her on Mother's Day, and she would say, Are you having a wonderful day with your wonderful family? Answer choices: Yes or No. How can you answer "No" to that question? Even if (1) your family has never been much for celebrating Mother's Day, so the kids will check in by bedtime, but pretty much leave it at that, (2) you have actually been grading papers all day, and (3) it is snowing on freaking Mother's Day because you live in Minnesota? Yes. I'm having a wonderful day with my wonderful family.

Although it felt like forever, the terrible pause ended. She cried a little, and I cried a little, and she soon got back on her game and asked me a lot of questions, most of which I did not know the answers to, which is her superpower. I told her the details I did know, and while we talked, Ruby put her head in my lap so I could rub her ears, which were perfectly soft and lovely, like a sealskin purse. I'm sure they have magical healing qualities.

We talked for just a few minutes, because you can't really talk about the weather and the flowers after that conversation, then we hung up so I could call my sisters and get the next part over with. But in the spirit of insuppressible optimism, she called me back a few hours later to tell me she had read online that if the cancer was Stage Zero, the survival rate was one hundred percent. Clearly, nothing to worry about.

Next, I called my sisters: Jane, Ann, and Ruth. Everyone should have three sisters, at least if they are sisters like mine. I am the baby, so that complicates things sometimes, when fifty years of family system mentality kicks in, and I forget that I'm a grown up and can actually drive the car or decide the menu, I don't have to let them do it and then get mad at them for doing it.

Jane offered advice, Ann offered to come help whenever I needed her, Ruth asked good questions and took it all in. In other words, they were all wonderfully themselves. And I didn't cry too much, even though I'm the baby.

Tier One: Mission Accomplished, more or less, by noon. I didn't call Jeff's mother, Sharon, to spread the news to his family. When I'm in a crisis and she is nice to me, I melt into a useless puddle on the floor. I decided to wait until I could get the words out of my mouth without sobbing. Maybe by tomorrow, I would have enough practice saying "I have cancer" that I would be able to get through those three words without losing it.

I spent the afternoon thinking about the Tier Two email and taking a nap, covers pulled over my head once again. Jeff hovered, trying to figure out what he could do for me and dealing with his own fears about what this would mean for our life together.

But that evening, I moved on to Tier Two. Another Mary-friend (I have five friends named Mary who played significant roles in my life at this time. What were parents thinking in the early Sixties?) had been diagnosed with breast cancer a couple of years earlier, and had sent out a lovely email informing friends, subject line "A Bump in the Road." I decided to follow her lead without borrowing her exact words.

I did not entitle my email "A Bump in the Boob," although I was tempted.

I took my time writing the email, then sat on the sofa with the computer on my lap, watching forgettable TV. I waited until the show was over, until just before bedtime, so I could go to bed and not look at my email the rest of the night. Then I hit "send."

About ten minutes later, the doorbell rang. I went to answer it, expecting it to be a friend of Sam's, because who else would be at our door at 10 p.m.? But there stood my friend Carolyn, one of my favorite people in the whole world. Over the years, we have cried together about our domestic frustrations, traveled together to Italy, and generally relied on each other to witness life's highs and lows. She lives about a block away.

She had gotten my email, walked right out of her house, bee-lined to my door, and rung the bell. She did not say anything, because, really, there was nothing to say. She stepped into the foyer, took me in her arms, held me a long time, then turned and left.

Although I would not have been able to tell you this ahead of time, that was exactly what I needed to wrap up this first day of my life with cancer.

•   •   •   •   •

In the months and years after my diagnosis, I resisted learning lessons from cancer. Starting from the day of my diagnosis, I concluded over and over again that cancer meant nothing about me or about my life. It was not a message to shape up. It was not something I deserved. I did not create it with negative thoughts. And I know it was not caused by, or even predicted by, unconnected events like falling down as I made my way in the world, even though I have those thoughts and must resist their pull. It was just something that happened. Much as I wanted to have control over this beast blocking my path, I didn't.

But with each step along this winding path, I learned that even if the fact of cancer meant nothing, how the people in my life responded to cancer, and how I received that response, meant everything. Our human connections, our care and tending to each other in the face of random, meaningless events—that's what we have in life. That's what sustains us. That's what matters.

And there, standing barefoot on the cool tile of my front foyer on a warm summer night, in my friend's arms, moths flitting around the porch light, a spark of illumination flared.

•   •   •   •   •

Being a Parent with Cancer puts you in a difficult spot, especially if your habitual mode of parental operation has been to over-protect your kids while knowing intellectually the whole time that it's the wrong approach. Which is pretty much the story of my generation's parenting.

I've had my reasons for over-protecting my kids, as do we all. I want them to feel special and supported, to experience only smooth sailing, to achieve the success I know they are capable of. As the youngest in a family of four girls, I decided at an early age that I was not so special, and if I needed anything out of life, I would have to make it happen on my own.

I don't mean to fault, my parents. Life was different in the America of the 1950s and 60s. As part of the Cold War effort, I guess, families had a lot of kids, most of whom were sent out the door at 8 a.m., vibrating from their Cap'n Crunch and Tang, and not expected to darken that screen door again until dinnertime. That's just how it was. No one was worried about serial killers or childhood self-esteem or getting a start on the Harvard application before kindergarten.

This generational attitude is illustrated by the great tragic-humorous story of my childhood, the story my father told about my birth pretty much every chance he got. The day I was born, he reported, he went over to the hospital at 10 o'clock at night. At the nursery window, the nurse held me up for inspection and said, Isn't she beautiful?

I've got three more at home just like her, he replied.

Then he turned around and went home.

Like I said, I don't fault my father. (Well, okay—a little.) I think this was actually his way of saying how much he loved all four of us and was proud to be our father. The times were just different. We're messed up in other ways now. But, having taken away the message that I was not so special and pretty much on my own, I swore I would never give my children the opportunity to draw the same painful conclusion.

As a parent, I have come to understand that children actually *need* to draw these conclusions—but maybe to a lesser extent than I did. They are special, but not too special. They do need to make it on their own, but we will support them as they struggle. And some terrible things will happen to them, many of which you can neither protect them from nor help them with very much. Crohn's Disease and cancer, for instance.

Anyway, I had to decide how to tell my children, Sam and Elena, that their mother had cancer. I think I did it wrong in both instances.

With Sam, I went with Casual. As if it would not impact his life at all or really matter very much to him.

Around five o'clock that Saturday, between the Tier One calls and the Tier Two email, after I'd had my nap, Jeff and I were standing around the kitchen island, tending to the household business, which, I was starting to learn, goes on despite cancer. We were sorting the mail and checking in about the day. Has the dog been walked? Did the cat pee on the floor today? Did anyone step in it? Did you notice if the lawn guy showed up yesterday? Are noodles okay for dinner?

Sam breezed in from his latest adventure, trailing the perfume of summer air, and tossed his scooter helmet on the counter. He went directly to the fridge, poured himself some orange juice, then started putting cream cheese on a bagel.

Yes, I said to Jeff. Noodles are fine for dinner.

By the way, I said to Sam, I have breast cancer. Did I get the right kind of cream cheese?

Sam looked up from his bagel, confused. Oh my gosh, Mom.

I'm fine. It will be fine. I'll probably have a little surgery next week, and that will be it. It's early. It can't be much cancer. You don't need to worry about it. I just want you to know.

Sam stammered a few questions and told me he was sorry. But I rushed on to ask what his plans for the evening were and how his work schedule was shaping up for next week.

Don't worry about little old me, honey. I expect nothing from you.

This was totally the wrong approach, not only because Sam is a thoughtful, sensitive guy who loves his mother, and it completely short-changed him. But also because it sent him the message that it wouldn't matter to *me* if he disengaged from the whole painful situation. Of course it mattered to me. But I am not so special, and I am on my own, so I would not want to admit that.

I handled the conversation with Elena little better. We waited all weekend, not sure whether to tell her or not. But Sunday afternoon, her cousin posted a vague reference to my news on Facebook, and we realized it would be terrible to have Elena find out that her mother had cancer from Facebook.

So Sunday night, I called her. I should not have called her. I don't know why I thought it would be okay to call her. She was away, after all, but only six blocks away. I should have gone to see her. It seems so obvious now.

My thinking was that I didn't want to disrupt her summer camp experience, which in retrospect is completely ridiculous. Her mother had cancer. By definition, her summer camp experience was about to be disrupted. It's not like we were going to wait two weeks until she got home to tell her, when everyone else in the world would know by then. Or that calling, not going in person, would make the news less painful.

It became clear when Elena started to hyperventilate on the phone that we should walk the six blocks to see her in person, so we did. It was a moonless summer night, but the stars blinked above us, so far away. We stood in the middle of the college quad, and I held her while she sobbed. Jeff patted us both on our backs. Pat pat. Pat pat. In this moment, I'm not sure how, but I managed not to cry myself. Elena was only sixteen at the time, and she needed me to be strong.

Much as I wanted to make it better for her, and as many times as I repeated that I would be fine, we would get through this, she would be okay, I realized in that moment: you can't take care of your kids forever. In fact, when you're girding your own loins for the epic battle ahead, you have to decide: someone else will need to help her deal with this. As much as I want to be a perfect, selfless, ever-supportive parent, not only is that impossible in general, but cancer is not going to let me. I will need to put everything I've got into the fight. That is what's best for her.

And in fact, that night, I took the first step down that road: letting someone else take care of it. I would get more practice with this later. Letting people bring me meals. Letting people drive me places. Letting people empty my surgical drains and clean up my vomit. Letting people just sit with me to keep me company. I have never been very good at any of this, but I got better.

We left Elena at her dorm and headed home. But I later learned that she called her friend Casey, who came over and took her away from summer camp, where she struggled to swallow the hard biscuit of this news, and wrapped her in a quilt, and fed her comfort food, and kept her overnight.

All without me. Which is how it had to be.

Chapter Three

Once the word is out that you have cancer, two things happen. One: you have to get down to the business of having cancer. Which actually takes a lot of time. If only you could earn a living putting in all those hours. (Wait a minute ...) Two: you have to deal with being guilty of Having Cancer in Public.

The main symptom of Having Cancer in Public is a lot of eye avertings. It begins with the mammogram technicians on the day you are diagnosed and spreads like an Asian swine-bird super virus. You go to Target because you need cat litter and Craisins, and you can't escape the feeling that the aisles are clearing in front of you as you push your cart to the back of the store where the pet supplies are shelved. It's like Moses and the Red Sea. Isn't that Jennifer Smith? Hi Jennif— And she's around the corner and down the shampoo aisle before you can get the words out.

Of course, this is because people just don't know what to do in an aisle at Target when confronted with the physical manifestation of human mortality. Especially people who did not hear the news directly from you, but heard it from their neighbor, who heard it from the cashier at the co-op, who heard it from your husband's colleague, who etc., etc. You don't know if they know, and they don't know if you know that they know, and you don't know if they know that you know that they know, and so on. This has to go on for a couple of weeks before everyone can assume that everyone knows, and then it's polite for them to just ask how your treatment is going and you can say *fine*, and you can both skip the whole "sorry you have cancer" thing. This is what manners are for.

Besides, they just went to Target because *they* needed cat litter and Craisins, and they really just want to get their errands done and go home. And who can blame them? I'm the same way.

But then there are the people you run into who clearly don't know. Friends, but not quite First Tier friends, so they didn't get the memo about your diagnosis you sent to *those* friends a few days back, and they are at Target because they just got back into town from a two-week vacation and there is literally no food in the house, so they have not talked to anyone yet. These people bring the cart to a complete stop, put on a friendly smile, and say, I haven't seen you in forever! How are you?! You look great!

Fine? Or not fine? That is the question.

If you choose fine, then later, when they find out you were in fact not fine, they will feel foolish and terrible, and it will be your fault. If you choose not fine and deliver the news right there, they will feel foolish and terrible in the middle of Target, and it will be your fault.

If only Miss Manners would weigh in.

Then there are the complete strangers who take their customer service jobs way too seriously, maybe because they earn a five-dollar Starbucks gift card if someone says something nice about them to the manager. Case in point: the clerks at Macy's.

The clerks at Macy's go out of their way to ask actually pretty invasive questions, like: So what have you been up to this morning? What kind of day are you having? What are your plans for this beautiful weekend?

I don't know who trains them to do this. I'd prefer they keep it to a smile and a basic, how are you? It bothers me under even normal circumstances. Under normal circumstances, I smile and say "fine," "not much," "yes" or "no", because I was not raised in a barn. But I get a little passive aggressive about it when, to tell you the truth, my afternoon has been pretty awful because I just had an extremely awkward breast MRI to determine whether my cancer is as extensive as my doctor suspects it might be. So I am guilty of giving the clerk at Macy's way more than she bargained for when she asked how my day was going.

All this social navigation is exhausting, and there really is no preparation for it. You could choose to stay home and avoid everyone. But really, what's the point of that? Cancer does not change the essential you, and everyone around you needs to get that message. You still have to go out there and buy the cat litter and change it when you get home besides. You can still laugh and chat in the aisle and care about the upcoming school musical. Just be ready to look people in the eye, speak from your heart, and be the courageous person you have always been. At least as best you can.

•   •   •   •   •

So starting on Monday of that next week, I had all this social navigation to tend to, but I also had to start the medical spanking machine. Remember in the good old days, before spanking was considered abusive and communal butt touching was not grounds for academic expulsion? When you had to go through the spanking machine at school on your birthday? All the kids in the class would line up in two rows, facing each other, and the birthday child would have to crawl through the middle while everyone whacked them on the butt as hard as they could and as many times as they could. The mean boys would use a social studies book as a paddle. Ahh, the Sixties.

The week after my diagnosis felt something like that. But with doctors.

I really wanted to get this started because I still thought it was just a tiny bit of cancer that would be taken care of in a few weeks, and a bad summer cold lasts about that long, so no problem. I'd be back at work in no time.

So on Monday, I waited a few hours to hear from the nurse at the clinic, who was supposed to set me up with The Next Step, because I did have the presence of mind to remember that my doctor was going to be out on Monday, but she would ask the nurse to get me going. I waited until about 11 a.m., then called and explained politely that I was diagnosed with cancer on Friday, and I was waiting to get set up for The Next Step, and could they please make sure the nurse called me back. Then I waited until about two o'clock and called again, and said I was so sorry to be a pest, but I was just a little anxious, and would they make sure the nurse got my message. Then I called at about 4:30 and said, I know you close at five, SO WHAT THE F**K IS GOING ON?

At about 5:15, the breast cancer coordinator (another surprise—there is so much breast cancer out there, it needs a coordinator) called me back and apologized for the delay, but said they had had some technical difficulties. Which was code for, the nurse screwed up. Anyway, she had gotten me set up for an appointment on Wednesday at the Piper Breast Center in Minneapolis. Was that okay? Well, it's not tomorrow, which it might have been if SOMEONE had actually taken care of it this morning, so it will probably shave a few days off my life. But I didn't have much choice at that point. So yes. That's okay.

Spanking number one.

Let me be clear. I don't mean to fault the medical practitioners who cared for me over these many months. I can't imagine the fortitude it takes to work with despairing cancer patients day after day. For the most part, the medical practitioners, especially the nurses, who cared for me were unfailingly kind, compassionate, and knowledgeable. I could even excuse that first nurse in my primary care clinic. She was just young, and probably afraid of me because she was supposed to call me to talk about cancer when she was more used to calling patients to talk about prescription refills.

In fact, who my nurses were became much more important in some ways than who my doctors were. You choose doctors who are highly educated experts, and who can wield a knife skillfully or make good decisions about what chemotherapy you need and how much. And the system has already vetted them pretty well for those qualities. Yes, you have to be able to work with their personalities, and some of them are more willing to explain themselves and talk about options than others. But for me personally, there is a broad range of "acceptable" out there, maybe because I usually research my questions ahead of time, so I go in mostly knowing what the story is and not asking the doctor to explain much. And maybe because I am fortunate enough to live in Minnesota, a state that offers some of the best health care in the world, and I have Cadillac insurance that allows me to go anywhere I want for treatment.

But the difference between evaluating doctors and evaluating nurses is kind of like the difference between buying a car and buying a bed. When you're buying a car, you need to think about safety and performance and gas mileage and potential repair costs. There are statistics on those things, and you can look them up on the Internet. Style and comfort may be more or less important to you, and there are individual lemons, but lots of cars out there will get you where you need to go day after day without killing you or leaving you stranded on the side of the road.

But when you're buying a bed, you need to think about what it's going to feel like when you sink into it every night. Supportive, yet pillowy? Or cavernous and lumpy? They may all look about the same, but your back knows that the cheap-ass one is going to make your life miserable. And there are no statistics to help you gauge quality.

With cancer, the nurses are what you sink into every night. You call them when you're so nauseated you can't eat, when you have yet another urinary tract infection resulting from your treatment, and when you are terrified about the test results that have not arrived yet. I am very grateful that good and dedicated people, who could probably make more money doing something else, choose to devote themselves literally around the clock to taking care of people like me.

•   •   •   •   •

The next day, Tuesday, I went to work and tried to be normal, thinking I would avoid the spanking machine for a day. Late summer in an academic institution is kind of like London during the plague. Only the die-hards and crazy people are around. So I could hole up in my office, sneaking out to go to the ladies room every few hours, and it actually would be fairly normal.

But about ten o'clock, I got a call from the breast clinic. They wanted me to come in for a breast MRI so they could get more information than the mammograms and biopsies had given them about the extent of my cancer. I had never heard of a breast MRI, so this did not seem like good news. And extent? What extent? I had just a tiny bit of cancer. Left breast. About seven o'clock.

They could get me in at one o'clock that day.

A breast MRI is very weird. You lie on your stomach on a cold, hard table, naked from the waist up (there was going to be a lot of naked from the waist up in the next few weeks) wondering if your neck can take another minute of this, while your breasts hang down into little pits so they can be zinged with MRI lightsaber beams. This is not a position you assume for any other purpose in your life, although I have to admit to a limited imagination in some arenas, and is certainly not the favorite pose for a forty-something-year-old woman who is all too aware of just how saggy and depleted her previously nice, firm breasts have become in the last ten years. In fact, it's quite humiliating. But okay. One for the team.

And as with most of these procedures, you have to hold very still and not breathe for several seconds every time they shoot the lightsabers at you. But at least these techs are so used to cancer patients that they don't bat an eye at your humiliation or your distressing condition. No eye averting. Just down to business, all in a day's work. I actually was pretty grateful for that.

The MRI took about an hour. Afterward, my neck was sore, and my energy was depleted. I made my way back to the parking garage, a route that would become all too familiar over the next several weeks. This is the bathroom I would stop in every day. This is the level I would park on. This is where I would turn left to get back to the highway, so I could drive not back to work, but home once again, where I could climb into bed and escape for a few hours into a dreamless sleep.

•　　　•　　　•　　　•　　　•

Several days after the MRI, I pulled a letter from my insurance company from the stack of mail on the kitchen counter. My stomach fluttered as I slid a knife into the corner of the envelope and eased it across the top. I pushed away the cat, who batted at the fold of white paper as I pulled it from the envelope and shook it open. I had great insurance, Cadillac insurance, but I dreaded learning that some expensive procedure would not be covered, that the treatment decisions were not mine to make, that I suddenly owed $10,000, the cost of one more stop in the spanking machine.

The letter granted post hoc approval for the MRI, deemed a "discretionary procedure." As if the MRI were a little extra add-on, like champagne in the room upon arrival. I read it through twice, just to make sure.

I had no complaints about my insurance company during this ordeal. They never balked at the bills for my treatment, and I never had to descend into that living hell of phone menus and petty bureaucracy that many cancer patients experience. But that letter made me realize that some of my treatment decisions were not mine to make, at least not realistically. If the insurance company took it into their corporate heads that a procedure was unnecessary, then I would probably not have it, no matter what my doctors recommended. Or at least I would not have it without some amount of delay, hassle, anguish, and argument.

I'm pretty sure that my thirty-minute MRI cost more than I make in a month, which was sobering. It was even more sobering when, over the next many months, I began to add up the bills as they came in and realized that the cost of my entire course of treatment could bankroll a minor coup in a small island nation. Throw the Crohn's Disease treatment into the family medical bill mix, and you've got enough for two minor coups or one really big one.

I suppose someone needs to keep tabs on whether expensive tests like MRIs are reasonably necessary under the circumstances, or medical costs would be even crazier than they already are. But as I stood in my kitchen reading that letter, I felt keenly the privilege of Cadillac health insurance. I remembered the twinge of guilt, the ping of discomfort at my own good luck, that I'd felt when passing badly copied fliers for a spaghetti dinner at the VFW or a pancake breakfast at the Lutheran church, orchestrated to fund cancer treatment for John Smith or Suzy Jones. Sure, I would sometimes stuff a few bucks in the donations jar at the coffee shop or send a small check after a community tragedy. But it never felt like enough.

As I read the letter, relieved that I would not spend my diminishing energy on an insurance appeal, or need to refinance the house to pay the bills, the financial and practical reality of cancer treatment hit me. And I wondered: How many people find themselves in cancerland without the resources to hack away at the jungle? How do people cope? Wouldn't financial insecurity and family stress make cancer a hundred times worse?

I haven't lived that story, so I can only guess at the answers. I can only tell my own story—about how I coped. But in telling my story, I am acutely aware of the privilege, financial and otherwise, that cushioned my life during cancer. In addition to excellent health insurance, I had a supportive family, a flexible job, and access to the best health care in the world. My friendships were deep and wide, and my friends were generous and kind. My family and friends are financially secure and also have flexible jobs, so they could tend to me without risking their own material well-being. I could afford to eat fresh, organic food, to try crazy supplements that may or may not have helped, to go for acupuncture and massage. I have time in my life to exercise.

I also live in one of the best small towns in America—literally, number two, if you choose to believe U.S. News and World Report. I am safe here, and the pace of life is moderate for the twenty-first century. It's clean, and you can hear the birds sing and the wind in the trees. People ride bikes and walk. They talk to each other on the street and in the coffee shop. There is poetry pressed into the concrete sidewalk every few blocks. The signs welcoming you to town sum it up: Cows, Colleges, and Contentment.

I know that most people who suffer with cancer are not so fortunate. For many, cancer takes a huge financial toll. They struggle with health insurance and with paying the household bills. They simply cannot work during treatment, or their employers are not-so-understanding. Or they live in places in the world where they are not safe, or they can't drink the water, or cancer treatment cannot be a priority. And cancer can scare people away, rather than bring them closer. It can strike when you are mostly alone in the world or overcome by family stresses or vulnerable in so many other ways.

I know I am lucky to have such a rich life, good fortune buoying me in so many ways. But at the same time, I can't discount my experience because it occurred in a context of privilege. It was still terrible and traumatic. In the eighteen months following my cancer diagnosis, I suffered physically and thought constantly about whether I would survive. The fact is, when it comes down to it, we are, all of us, mortal beings who feel pain and don't want to die. Privilege may provide more resources to cope with that basic reality, but it does not take it away.

Because of who I am and how I'm positioned in the world, my story cannot be everyone's story. Of course, that will be true for anyone's crisis story. I try to remember that each story is important. Each story is unique. Each story contributes to the vast cosmos that is human experience.

·   ·   ·   ·   ·

The next day, Tuesday, when I had the Big Appointment at the breast center, to see first a surgeon then a radiologist, it became clear that the MRI films were crucial to a good diagnosis.

Jeff went with me to the Big Appointment that day. Jeff is my husband, and he loves me, and I had just been diagnosed with cancer. So of course he wanted to come with me, even if he'd be stranded in the first of many pink waiting rooms all day, listening to soothing music and refusing beverages from the touchingly eager volunteers. But if I allowed Jeff to put his busy life on hold for the day, it upgraded the crisis, making it bigger than I wanted it to be. It meant I actually had cancer.

As we got ready to go that morning, I had to resist the urge to say, no, no—I can do this on my own. I'll be fine. You don't need to come. I swallowed those words dozens of times as Jeff packed up his computer, poured iced tea into our travel cups, and propelled me out the door to the car, where he slid behind the wheel so I could stare out the window as the rows of corn sped by.

I have come to understand that telling people who love you that you don't need them, that they shouldn't come along, is actually a kind of selfishness. The people who love you want to help. You are part of their lives, so this is their experience too. They need to be involved, to experience their feelings, so they can process their own grief, alongside yours. Besides, you *don't* have to do it on your own, and insisting that you do diminishes a fundamental joy of being alive: both giving *and* receiving generosity and love. Although I only later fully understood this, early in my cancer experience I began to realize that I should keep these words—no, I can do this on my own; no, I don't need help—from coming out of my mouth.

Say yes, I told myself. Say yes to the world. Say yes to everyone.

This was hard for me, and I needed practice. Today was an opportunity to practice.

But it was not an easy day to practice. Cancer is inconvenient. It does not wait politely for your calendar to clear so you can attend to it. It does not ask permission. It ambushes, and you have no choice but to drop what you are doing and pay attention.

Jeff and Sam had tickets to fly to Indianapolis later that day for Geekfest America, also known as GenCon. GenCon was THE big gaming convention in the U.S., where people (read: male people) spend several days in malodorous rooms playing Magic the Gathering while wearing Klingon costumes. Sam has always been a big gamer, even though he is way too cool for Klingon costumes, and Jeff loves games too, although he's too old and too responsible to immerse himself in gaming culture the way Sam does. The two of them had road-tripped to the convention every year since Sam was about ten, while Elena and I stayed home to clean closets, then reward ourselves with chick-flick marathons fueled by pints of Ben and Jerry's.

So it worked for Jeff to come to the appointment with me this morning, but the schedule was tight. He needed to be at the airport with Sam by late afternoon. If all went as planned—consult with the surgeon, check in with the radiologist, have a treatment plan in place by noon— this would be no problem. But I was nervous.

We arrived at the breast center early and were quickly settled into an exam room. I took out my book, and Jeff opened his laptop and connected to the clinic's wi-fi. The clinic décor was understated, tending towards pink, but with plenty of blue and green to balance it out. The robes were cozy, the lighting was warm, and tea was available around every corner. Everything was muted, cushiony, carefully chosen to help you absorb this blow to your life plan.

We met first with a nurse, whose job it was to get my whole story. I am unreasonably proud that I can rattle off medical terms like ablation and dermoid cyst during my medical history review without stumbling. There is a reason why, among all the commercial cancer junk on the market out there, you can buy a button that says "nurses favorite." (Yes, the one I was given is missing the apostrophe, because when it comes to cancer, all rules, even grammatical ones, are suspended.) Later, I discovered that relating this history every time you sit down in an exam room gets tedious. In fact, in my years since cancer, I find myself just leaving details out because it all feels so tedious. But this nurse was patient and truly wanted all the details. When she reached the end of her questions, she patted my hand, stood to leave, and told me the doctor would be in soon.

Next into the room: Dr. Ryan, the surgeon. It doesn't seem quite fair that the doctor you spend the least time with, in all this cancer mess, at least while conscious, the surgeon, actually has some of the harder jobs: (1) taking the first stab at explaining everything that is likely to happen to you in the next six months or a year, when you are still reeling emotionally from the diagnosis, and (2) delivering all the bad news, before and after surgery, other than the initial bad news that you already know.

Despite my claim that I usually do my research ahead of time and can tolerate a range of doctor personalities, I had not done a lot of research before this appointment. I was thinking, get in there, get it over with, get back to work. I got set up with a reputable surgeon at a reputable clinic connected to a reputable hospital, and I forged ahead. Make sure the water is deep enough, then close your eyes and jump. I did ask a few friends in the medical profession if they had recommendations, or had heard anything about this surgeon, and it appeared that the water was in fact sufficiently deep. So I jumped.

And I got lucky. Dr. Ryan was excellent, and he took a huge amount of time explaining the options and procedures to us. He drew pictures, wrote down notes, made recommendations, and pointed us to web sites. He told us that his colleagues over in plastic surgery were doing some really great work with reconstruction. He was thinking that a lumpectomy (left side, seven o'clock) would do the trick, and we could maybe even get that on the schedule for Friday, before he left for vacation next week. He would have his assistant take a look at his schedule.

I sat back in my chair, relieved. If I could have a lumpectomy on Friday, I thought, this would all be over within a few weeks, before school started again for me, even. Yes, Jeff would be in Indianapolis with Sam on Friday, but by happy circumstance, not good planning, since cancer accommodates only chance, not planning, my sister Ann was coming to town on Thursday just for a visit. She could shepherd me through the surgery, and Jeff would be home on Sunday. This cancer thing had been inconvenient, but not that big a deal. I totally had this under control.

I smiled at Jeff. Sounds like a good plan, huh? I said.

He frowned, not happy about the idea that I would have the surgery without him there as support. But Ann was coming, and that was the next best thing. So it could probably work.

Over the next half-hour, though, it became clear that something wasn't going according to plan. Dr. Ryan left the room several times to check on the radiologist, who was looking at the MRI films. Then he would come back into the room and say, oh she's not quite finished with that yet, and keep talking, drawing another diagram or offering more details about tumor types. Then he would get up and leave again, door whooshing shut behind him.

As we waited and Dr. Ryan went in and out of the room, I got the impression that there were technical difficulties of some sort, but I wasn't worried. Lumpectomy on Friday, I thought. Thank goodness. Let's get this over with.

I didn't yet understand that I was the technical difficulty.

After several comings and goings, Dr. Ryan finally came in to stay. He sat down, pulled his chair close, and looked me in the eye. I became aware of the cold blasting from the air conditioning. I pulled my cushiony robe close and did my best to meet his gaze.

The radiologist is still reading the films, he said, and she has some concerns. The MRIs suggest that we should do some additional biopsies. Can you stick around for the afternoon? That will help us get a better idea of what is going on. We're not sure yet what this means.

He was well trained not to eye-avert because he is a surgeon. But I could feel those neurons firing overtime, signaling his eye muscles that they must hold firm. All hands on deck. He held my gaze.

I looked away, out the window at the HVAC equipment on the roof next door. Hot sun glinted off the metal ductwork, blinding me.

It was just before noon. We'd been at the clinic for almost three hours. Jeff's flight was at five o'clock.

I knew we were in exactly the kind of impossible position cancer puts you in. If we stayed for the afternoon, for more imaging, we would soon have to decide. Should Jeff stay home with me for the next leg of the spanking machine? Because who knew what this afternoon's images would show, and whether I could actually have a quick lumpectomy on Friday, with Ann here to hold my hand? Or should he fly to Indianapolis with Sam, his chronically ill son, for the annual dose of increasingly precious father-son bonding time, which could end any year now that Sam was moving into adulthood?

I turned to look at Jeff. He needed to pack. I had work planned for the afternoon. And the dog would need her walk.

Jeff took my hand and nodded. Of course, he said. We can stick around. We'll walk next door and get some lunch. Whatever it takes. When do you need us back?

They'll be ready for you at about one, Dr. Ryan said. It may take several more hours. I'm sorry.

After Dr. Ryan left the room, I tossed the cushy robe and blue and white hospital gown in a corner and pulled on my civilian clothes. I threw open the exam room door and elbowed my way through the throng of the pink-scrubbed nurses gathering their lunch bags and purses, Jeff keeping pace behind me. In the elevator, I held back my tears, thinking about how many tears that elevator had probably seen. We exited the elevator, and I followed Jeff through the maze of hospital buildings and skyways to the nearby global marketplace.

At the market, we managed to choke down some food and tried to talk about our options. But the noise and commotion of people going about their routine, everyday lives were disorienting. How could the world continue so normally, when we were in such crisis? We headed back towards the hospital, but ended up sitting on the floor in an empty beige corridor, hung with pictures documenting the hospital's history. Jeff got on the phone with the airline and tried to figure out a plan, while I stared at the pictures, my back against the cool, concrete wall, wondering how many families had sat in this grim corridor before me, trying to see the future.

Airlines are completely forgiving when it comes to death, even though it is so, well, flexible after the fact. But they are not so forgiving when it comes to immediate medical crises happening in the location you are in. When my father died, I got a special rate on the next plane out of Minneapolis, even though he was already gone, and my getting there quickly would do neither of us any good. And if I had had a medical crisis in Indianapolis, Jeff would have gotten a great rate to come be with me. But he was not able to convince the airline to change his flight to the next day, even on standby, so that he could *stay* in the city where I was actually *having* the medical crisis. It made no sense.

We decided Sam should fly out without him, and we would just wait to see what happened next. Then we returned to the clinic, where Jeff was consigned to yet another pink waiting room, while I was ushered back into another dimly lit procedure room, for my mystery date with radiologist number two.

Besides the date night lighting, these procedure rooms are notable for the ceilings. This room, like many that would follow, had special ceiling features designed to supply visual interest for the patient strapped to the table. Or at least a distraction. Sometimes, as in this room, it was just regular ceiling tiles painted with unusual colors and patterns to jazz things up. Sometimes it was an inspirational poster, or a child's drawing in primary colors, or an origami mobile.

These efforts are well intentioned. Hang in there, baby. When life gives you lemons, make lemonade. Life is short; eat dessert first. (Wait. That one would be really tactless, so that probably didn't happen.) Those ceiling tiles were one link in a long chain of efforts people made to calm my fears and assuage my pain. But colorful ceiling tiles don't go far to assuage the pain of lying there, staring up into the indifferent grey sky, wondering about the meaning of your life. On the other hand, many other efforts, large and small, made by a multitude of people who stood by me during this time, did help. And in fact, carried me across that raging river. So I guess I can't pick on the ceiling tiles, because in some sense, all those efforts accumulated over time. I have to appreciate every one of them, no matter the magnitude.

I assumed the position, flat on my back, naked from the waist up but for the paper clinic gown, while the radiologist explored the local terrain with the ultrasound wand. This time, it was both breasts, because apparently the MRI had shown "areas of concern" on both sides. This explained all the coming and going from the exam room and why the morning session had taken so long. I was one big technical difficulty.

In fact, there were so many areas of concern, on both sides, they couldn't quite decide where to send the blue crab with the pinchers for sampling. The radiologist took some pictures, then stepped out to look at them. She came back and took more pictures, then stepped out to look again. At some point in the next forty-five minutes, a technician or nurse came in (I couldn't tell them apart at this point) and said: you have very active breasts.

I thought: Maybe in high school. But if you want to know the truth, they have not been all that active in the last few years, peri-menopause, work stress, teenagers in the house, and all. But that's middle age for you.

Then I thought: Very active breasts? What the hell?

What they meant: I had cancer everywhere. On both sides. Ultimately, every single one, two, three THWACK from that afternoon came up cancerous. The radiologist stopped at about a dozen. I went home feeling like I'd been assaulted by a hyperactive eight-year-old making hole-punch confetti for the school play.

Thus began my course correction. This was not a tiny bit of cancer. It was not going to be Stage Zero. It was not going to be cleared up in a few weeks. This was going to take over my life for a while.

Crack.

•　　•　　•　　•　　•

We decided that Jeff should follow Sam to Indianapolis on Thursday because I would not have a lumpectomy that week, or any time soon. Nothing else could happen until those biopsies came back from the lab, determining the future of my very active breasts. The results would not be back until Friday afternoon.

Ann would arrive on Friday afternoon and stay until Monday morning. That meant I would not be alone during most of the next few days, and she would be able to keep me suited up for the basketball game and help me ignore the gorilla.

I resumed my routine for forty-eight hours. Walked the dog. Went to work. Ate my kale and yogurt. Did some yoga. Tried to stay positive and hope for the best. But during times like this, when I was waiting for news and couldn't help but be anxious, I felt suspended in midair, both present and not present. I watched small-town life proceed around me on its usual course and watched myself participate in it. Sweet corn and downtown band concerts. Trips to Target. Coffee in the morning, iced tea in the afternoon. But none of it felt real. My life did not stop, but it also could not move forward. Like a stick snagged on a rock mid-stream. It might stay stuck, current parting around it, for months. Or, with the right swell of current, it might suddenly dislodge and rejoin the flow, blithely on course for the next destination. I didn't know.

Friday afternoon, I went out to walk Ruby early, even though it was hot, she's extremely furry (even after she sheds two garbage bags worth of undercoat in June), and she hates the heat. Fortunately for her, we'd left the snout houses behind just a few months earlier in search of a more compatible neighborhood, and we now lived in the idyllic old part of town where mature trees are plentiful. She liked to zig-zag from shady spot to shady spot on those warm summer walks, and when she found one with just the right amount of cool still hiding in the grass, she would dive in and roll around on her back, trying to soak up as much of it as she could. She did the same thing in the snow in winter, and could find the last remaining patch of snow in March (or May, as the case may be), even if it was barely enough to make a respectable snowball, so she could enjoy one more rapturous roll. Watching her do this was right up there on the list with Minnesota sweet corn in July.

I would have preferred not to get the phone call while out walking the dog because she was not very patient standing still, especially when it was hot. But I had my phone tucked into the pocket of my shorts where I could feel it buzz, in case a completely off-course semi drove down Maple Street and drowned out the ringtone, because I had to get the walk done so I could drive to the airport to pick up my sister. And of course, it rang when we were about six blocks from home, in an unshaded area of campus where there was no place to sit down.

Once again, my first reaction to bad news was to feel sorry for the doctor who had to deliver it. I'm sorry to put you in this miserable position. I know you are paid hundreds of thousands of dollars a year to do this job. And yet, I'm sorry.

But it was Friday afternoon again. And this doctor not only got to lock up and go home. He was heading out of town for vacation, probably to a luxury cabin on a private lake or to a villa in Italy.

Dr. Ryan explained that every biopsy had come back as cancerous. Ductal cancer, lobular cancer. You name it, I seemed to have it. They would not know the size of the largest tumor until they removed it and measured it during surgery, but there were at least several tumors on both sides. They couldn't say how many. My only choice was bilateral mastectomy. We'd have to wait and see about chemotherapy and radiation. An oncologist would probably want to do a CT scan and maybe some other tests to look for metastatic disease.

So I can't have a lumpectomy? I asked, as Ruby tangled herself up in an arborvitae, searching for a cool spot. You can't just take out these couple of tumors and get this over with next week?

He paused. No. You really need to have a bilateral mastectomy. Your cancer is quite extensive.

I know that in the next few minutes, I agreed that his assistant would set up an appointment with an oncologist to discuss whether I needed chemo before surgery, to shrink the tumors and increase the chance of a good result. I agreed that she would also set up an appointment with a plastic surgeon, so I could at least talk about options. I agreed that Dr. Ryan would check in on Wednesday next week, after I saw the oncologist, so we could decide whether to go ahead and schedule the surgery or proceed with chemo first. I agreed that I would call the breast clinic if I had questions.

I know I agreed to all of this, but I was not actually present for any of it. I was on my back, looking at the sky.

Somehow, Ruby and I walked the six blocks home, where my neighbor Laurie was out working in her yard. Laurie is a great neighbor, and I am very fond of her. But I had only lived across the street for a few months, and I made the same mistake I'd made with Samantha a week earlier. You're so overcome by this bag of rocks that just fell on you from the sky, you don't have good judgment about anything that happens in the next hour, or maybe the next year. So you tell this devastating news to someone who is not the right recipient. Laurie didn't deserve that. But she caught it gracefully anyway.

I went inside, released the dog to the basement, where she could find some relief on the concrete floor, and sat down in the breakfast nook. I needed to leave for the airport in about thirty minutes. But there was nothing to do. Any single thing I did in that moment seemed superfluous, mere theater. My body was busy marshaling all of my resources and sending them to the emotional processing portion of my brain, and even movement seemed impossible. I suppose it was shock.

I pulled myself together enough to call Carolyn, and miraculously, she was working at home that day. Once again, she bee-lined to my door and let herself in.

It seems ridiculous now that, despite my emotional state, I insisted I was fine to make the forty-five-minute drive to the airport to get my sister. Those childhood grooves (I'm fine, I can do it myself, don't trouble yourself about me) are both deep and wide, and especially in crisis, they are the default position. It takes everything you have to hoist yourself out of the rut and see reason.

Fortunately for me, Carolyn is both a wise person and a stellar friend. You know, she said, I am not one to tell you what to do. I will intervene only in extreme circumstances, when I know you are wrong. But these are those circumstances. You may not drive to the airport. I will drive you.

I let her drive. Say yes, I reminded myself, to everyone.

Chapter Four

Our brains crave patterns. We're pattern addicts. Patterns link us to cause and effect. Patterns plus cause and effect equal prediction. We want to predict: What next? So we ask: Why did this happen? And: What will happen next? A relentless quest to optimize happiness in the next moment. Or maybe just magical thinking.

I know that falling down three times and, consequently, striking out did not cause my cancer. That is just my brain, wanting a pattern fix.

I also know that dousing my clothes with bug repellant for a trip to northern Minnesota, where the state bird is the mosquito, two weeks before my diagnosis did not cause my cancer, although I joke about that a lot. Maybe all that Six-12 sprayed incontinently during childhood camping expeditions, but not the bug spray from last week. I'm also pretty sure that an unresolved disruption in my energy flow due to childhood trauma (you're not so special) did not cause my cancer. But I have not ruled that out as a contributing factor.

But when you go from clear mammogram to extensive invasive cancer, just like that, your brain really wants some answers. Without a story to tell yourself about how this happened, how can you possibly carry on? How can you feel any certainty about the prediction you must make when you climb out of bed every morning—the prediction that enables you to eat your vegetables and go to the job you're not so keen on anymore and continue to patch it up with your mate—that this is not your last day on earth?

People *want* to give you answers. The best doctors want to help you make sense of it. But they often don't know, not really. When I asked Dr. Ryan, the surgeon, what might have caused the extensive cancer it turned out I had, he fumbled. Maybe a virus, he said.

A virus, my ass. What, a boob virus? What about the creosote-polluted groundwater in the suburb where I spent my teens? What about the pesticides on the strawberries I picked during idyllic childhood summers at a mid-Ohio farm? What about the accidental gulps of Lake Erie I swallowed on camping trips down the shore from Cleveland, where the Cuyahoga River was burning as it flowed into the lake? What about the BPA in the plastic I heated my lunch in every day before I knew better? Each its own piece of ice, waiting to orchestrate my fall.

•　　　•　　　•　　　•　　　•

The medical gauntlet continued the following week, a regular full-time job. Agenda for Monday: appointment with Dr. Chen, the oncologist.

The first visit to the oncologist's office is terrifying because the waiting room is full of obviously very sick people with no hair, some of whom are attached to alarming medical devices. Their harried companions are busy making undrinkable powdered hot chocolate in Styrofoam cups and looking mournful. You think, is this going to be us in a month? Me in a bad paisley scarf and Jeff on hot chocolate duty? How can that be? I feel perfectly fine. I don't belong here.

Medical oncology made no emotional sense to me, at any point along the road, *because* I felt perfectly fine. My treatment took my apparently perfectly healthy body and mutilated, poisoned, and irradiated it, making it incredibly sick and unhappy, to no visible purpose. You can't see your breast cancer. Except for that weird grainy patch, I couldn't even feel it. I had to take Their word for it: I had cancer and quite a bit of it, and if I didn't act quickly, I might, apparently, die. This required a major suspension of disbelief, a project worthy of the greatest Hollywood talents. Even now, I have this niggling feeling that it was all made up, a ploy to accomplish some end that has yet to be revealed to me.

So I suspended my disbelief as Jeff and I trooped to the back of the clinic, which thankfully was not all pink, because they treat a veritable rainbow of cancers there, and were lodged in a small exam room with Bonnie.

Bonnie is one of the above-mentioned nurses, and Bonnie is a saint. Compassionate and knowledgeable, but able to maintain a sense of humor about the whole cancer thing. She also knew all the constipation remedies in the book, which is essential knowledge for a cancer nurse. When my first oncologist left the clinic for a new job: Whatever. When Bonnie moved to a different clinic, I moved with her. I would have moved into her basement if she'd let me. I sincerely hope she lives for a hundred years and her every dream comes true, because she deserves it. Like a dewy baby duck, I immediately imprinted on Bonnie.

The first question they ask you in an oncology exam, the question Bonnie started with when we got down to business, is: how much pain are you having today?

Well, my wrist was still a little sore from my January fall. And my neck has hurt since 1983. Did that count?

There again was that disbelief, ready for suspension. I had no pain. And I clung to my belief that I had done everything right. I had just spent a week up north hiking several hours a day. I had published a book that spring. Bonnie and I should be drinking herbal tea and talking about our kids, not discussing my pain or lack thereof.

So I told Bonnie I had no pain. We moved on to my exercise habits, my medications, and whether I felt safe at home. This question and answer session with Bonnie lasted about five minutes, and in the end, we determined that, except for that pesky cancer issue, I was very healthy.

Enter stage left: Dr. Chen. Dr. Chen seemed like a perfectly nice man, and he had stellar credentials as an oncologist. But he was a man of few words and no bedside manner. I felt like, to him, I was a chart and a dosage, dissociated from a body. Wasn't this whole ordeal about my body? But at that point, I was already in love with Bonnie (her husband plays mandolin in a bluegrass band, for heaven's sake), who seemed equipped to tell me everything I needed to know, and in the sincerest and most compassionate way. Besides, we were only there for an initial opinion about chemo before surgery or not.

Dr. Chen's opinion, in essence, was this: No. No chemo before surgery. But you need a CT scan. And a chest x-ray. Bonnie will arrange it. Come back Monday for results.

Exit stage left.

Bonnie patted me on the back, then patted Jeff on the back, then patted me on the back again, all the while saying reassuring things about how everything was going to be okay. She gave us lots of information about the CT scan, answered our few questions, and led us down the hall to the scheduling office.

• • • • •

At the Big Appointment the previous week, when Dr. Ryan told me what great work his colleagues over in plastics were doing with reconstruction, I was taken by surprise.

I did not begin that first week with breast cancer thinking about whether I valued my basic female form enough to contemplate multiple, potentially complicated surgeries that struck at the very core of my beliefs. But here I was, Tuesday of week two, and I found myself walking into yet another medical building for an appointment with a plastic surgeon.

The idea of plastic surgery and breast reconstruction had not even been on my radar until Dr. Ryan mentioned it, maybe because I was still in the "tiny bit of cancer" mindset, not in the bilateral mastectomy mindset. This seems like an egregious oversight on my part. There is, after all, a federal law, passed in 1998, that requires insurance companies to pay for breast reconstruction after mastectomy.

I am a lawyer. And a feminist. But I guess I was busy picking up Legos and making spaghetti in 1998, and I have the odd fortune to know very few women who have undergone mastectomies. Lumpectomies are more the norm, in my experience. It's a good example of how, no matter how well educated you think you are, sometimes you pay no attention until something is personally relevant to you.

I am actually rather judgmental about plastic surgery, especially when it comes to breasts. In college, I was the kind of feminist who decided: Damn the androcentric, classist, and racist female beauty industry! I won't conform to these ridiculous, sexist cultural ideals that doom women to anorexia and other bodily obsessions! I refuse to wear a bra! And I did refuse to wear a bra, for about ten years, until I was pregnant, when the gravity of my breasts threatened to tumble me into the gutter if they didn't have some shoring up.

Disdain for plastic surgery was an easy position for me since I live in a laidback Midwestern college town, where typical female attire is decent yoga pants, a fleece jacket over a turtleneck or t-shirt, and Birkenstocks or hiking boots, depending on the season. Actually, that's typical attire for men as well, maybe swapping out the yoga pants for jeans. Pierced ears are the fancy extra (both ears for women, one for men). When I started wearing mascara in 2007, because I noticed that I had pink rabbit eyes in the annual Christmas picture, I felt like a conspicuously painted woman.

Even now, I'm reluctant to probe my thinking about plastic surgery too deeply, probably because I fear that when it comes right down to it, I'm actually quite vain and have no principles. But I suppose I am like most people. Meaning, if you ask me to choose between donating money to starving children in Africa, who I don't know personally, and going on vacation, I go on vacation. Although maybe I make a larger contribution to UNICEF that month because of the guilt. So when I thought about years and years (I hoped!) of taking my shirt off at night and seeing only a flat, barren landscape in the mirror, I couldn't bear it (no pun intended).

But on the other hand, to be fair, I was only in my forties. In the previous five years, I had decided I wanted to look great in middle age, in a more conventional way than I had previously pursued. Call it a mid-life vanity crisis. Maybe a concession of youthful principles to the realities of aging. Maybe too much *What Not to Wear*, watched, in theory, to keep my feminist cultural analysis skills sharp.

In the couple of years before my diagnosis, I lost weight, started strength training, and threw out the baggy clothes that had accumulated in my closet after my kids were born. I had not had body image issues as a young woman. But I had not really embraced looking great either, whatever that meant, until recently. And suddenly, it seemed, I was going to be relegated back to hiding in clothing akin to flour sacks.

So I found myself walking down the dingy halls of a suburban medical office building, looking for the office of Dr. Smith. The fluorescent lights overhead dimly illuminated the faded salmon and turquoise, mid-eighties décor, which did not fit with my ideas about plastic surgeons' offices at all. The dreariness of the building made me feel a little better, because at least, apparently, I was not going to see a *swanky* plastic surgeon.

The office itself was somewhat cheerier, and the people were friendly, although they did not seem the least bit interested in my general health. I think in my two-year marathon of appointments in that office, they took my blood pressure twice (required by law, once a year). Ashley, Dr. Smith's assistant, was not a nurse (maybe a medical assistant), but she was always sweet and kind to me. More importantly for her job, perhaps, she was statuesque, well-dressed, and while not quite beautiful, knew how to create the illusion that she was. And she knew how to use a camera, which turns out to be an important qualification for a plastic surgeon's assistant.

Ashley ushered me into an exam room, told me to strip from the waist up, and handed me the most inadequate exam "gown" I had yet encountered: a disposable, pink bolero-type jacket. It went not quite to my waist, and the feel reminded me of the toilet paper in campground pit toilets. Maybe this was supposed to make me feel better about selling out to plastic surgery. No plush French terry robes here.

I waited on the plastic chair in the exam room for about ten minutes, shivering in my black linen capri pants, strappy sandals, and pink paper bolero jacket, for Dr. Smith to appear.

When Dr. Smith and Ashley swept into the room, I began to doubt my decision. Dr. Smith is a very handsome man. Let me say up front that he is also a wonderful and caring doctor, skilled and professional, and he took excellent care of me through some pretty rough times. But at first I thought he looked like a high-end huckster. Maybe a big-stakes gambler. Maybe the brains behind an international art heist. Too slick to be trusted. His suit was exceptionally well-tailored, and in a pinch, he could probably light the surgery suite with the shine on his wingtips. He also had great hair. My mind immediately jumped to Grey's Anatomy, and I wondered if the office supply closet got a lot of traffic.

I am not the only one to think this way. It was de rigueur that when Dr. Smith left a room, e.g., a surgical prep cubicle or a hospital room where I was confined to the bed, the next woman into the room would say: he's such a nice man. Which I believe was code for: my goodness, he's handsome. Even female doctors were compelled to say this. Post-menopausal female doctors. And when a colleague at work, who had just come through the breast cancer gauntlet herself, emailed me to say that Dr. Smith had been her surgeon, her first words were not "He's a great surgeon." They were "He's sure easy on the eyes!"

I found myself standing at attention, my pink paper wrapping having fallen to the floor, with a very handsome, slightly untrustworthy man in an expensive suit kneeling in front of me with a tape measure, inches from my sagging belly, measuring the width of my areolas and the distance between my navel and my breastbone. While he was down there, he also gauged some abdominal fat to see if it would suffice for natural tissue migration, an option instead of implants. When he announced that I did not have enough ab fat to make two replacement C cup breasts, I was relieved. At that point, you take your comfort where you can find it.

As the patient, what exactly are you supposed to do during this strange experience? Somehow, being examined standing up is worse than being examined lying down. At least lying down you can pretend that you are sick, and keep better tabs on the bolero jacket. And just where do you look? Do you look down at the doctor's very full head of hair? Do you look Ashley in the eye and make small talk? Do you close your eyes and think of England?

I chose eyes open, over my left shoulder, at the door. I stuck to that for the next two years.

Measuring complete, Dr. Smith helped me back into my so-called gown and sat down opposite me to talk through the options. I could have basic reconstruction, which could commence in the same surgery as the mastectomy and end, four surgeries later, with tattooing of areolas around artificially constructed nipples.

Or I could have the "lat flap" procedure, which would achieve a more "natural" look and feel. This procedure involves moving tissue and fat from your back and tacking it onto the front. So basically you end up with the same droopy breasts you started out with, except they are made from a different body part. This procedure was longer, riskier, and had a more difficult recovery time. But I did have enough back fat to make it possible. (Not enough belly fat, but enough back fat? Really? Couldn't he please take it from my butt instead, where fat was plentiful?) The nipple reconstruction and areola tattooing would then also be available, my choice.

I did not have to do any of this at the time of the mastectomy. These procedures would be available whenever I was ready, if that day ever came. I could do it now, or in ten years, whatever was right for me. The option was always available. I should go home and think about it.

Dr. Smith shook my hand, smiled his dazzling smile, and left the room.

Before I could go home and think about it, there was one last stop. Photos, courtesy of Ashley. The plastic surgeon's office has a special little room for photos. A darkened mugshot booth between the exam rooms, not unlike the arcade photo booth at the mall, but minus the smell and the sticky floor. I stood on the nubby rubber mat, matching my feet to the painted-feet outlines, pink paper jacket around my ankles, and followed Ashley's instructions.

Face me. A quarter turn to your right. Full turn to the right. Now a quarter turn to your left. Full turn to the left. Perfect. You can get dressed.

Many brave and compassionate women allow these photos to be posted on the Internet, so those of us wondering what dark road we're heading down can see the results for ourselves. I found these photos of other women to be quite heartening, because those colleagues over in plastics really are doing some amazing work. I became convinced, surfing breast reconstruction photos on the Internet, that if I went ahead with reconstruction, I would have the best boobs in the nursing home when I was eighty. For whatever that's worth.

The photos are generally anonymous, meaning the only mug involved is your chest; your face is excluded from the view. I understand the need for this singular focus on the breasts. Good breast reconstruction surgeons do their best to recreate your natural state, perhaps even resurrecting a younger-looking version, and your face is beside the point, and possibly distracting. But it's hard to put aside the feeling that your surgeon will remember you by your cup size, general flaccidity, and mole pattern rather than by your face, which is how we naturally want to be remembered.

In December 2012, when I was in Dr. Smith's office for my areola tattoos, the final stage of breast reconstruction, I saw these photos, taken during this first visit to Dr. Smith's office. The tattoo artist wanted to make sure she got the color right when she mixed the tattoo pigment. She gave me copies, which I now keep tucked away in my box of breast cancer mementos.

Looking at these photos over two years later, I cried for the first time in a long time. Although I cried plenty in the early weeks and months after my diagnosis, by 2012, I was pretty cried out, at least where cancer was concerned. But in these photos, there I was: my breasts. Naked, vulnerable, and anonymous. The part of me that had nourished my children and served me well all those years, harnessed or unharnessed. I had not been done with them, as a friend had suggested the week after my diagnosis, an ill-considered remark intended to make me feel better. I was actually quite attached to them, literally and figuratively. In the photos, I was covered with bruises and partially healed wounds, from all that thwacking and hole punching the week before. The photos looked like domestic violence evidence shots.

During the course of my treatment with Dr. Smith, Ashley took me into that little photo room and put me through my paces six or eight times. Those initial photos were the only ones I ever saw. But as I examined them, I imagined Dr. Smith, with his great hair and expensive suit, studying my photo gallery before each of my surgeries, gauging size and shape; lift and symmetry. Thinking about where to cut and paste.

How humiliating.

•   •   •   •   •

Wednesday spanking: CT scan and chest X-ray.

The CT scan and chest X-ray pronounce your sentence in the cancer tribunal: life, with some period of incarceration; probation, with a side of unpleasant community service; or death, with no chance of appeal, but maybe time for one last good meal. If the scans show that your bones and organs are clear, thumbs up. If a slight shading appears here, or a dark shadow there, thumbs down.

You never get to meet the person who reads these scans, the radiologist, who is too geeky to even invite you on this date; who is making the life or death call without you, in a dim room in the basement of the hospital. You never even know their name. You just get the bill: Consulting Radiologists, $457.86. Please remit to P.O. Box 1259, Oaks, Pennsylvania (why Pennsylvania?) 19456. It takes a lot of trust, I tell you.

The mundane experience of submitting to these scans is an odd counterweight to the magnitude of the results. I had these procedures in a major metropolitan medical facility, where I would have my mastectomy in a few weeks. People die there every day. But they are also born there every day. In fact, my son was born in that very hospital, twenty-one summers earlier. Many patients clearly much sicker than I were being wheeled in and out of the CT suite in gurneys and wheelchairs, or creeping down the hall with the help of walkers and canes. Some had bad backs from snow shoveling or tennis elbow. Others had metastatic cancer or end-stage heart failure. Luck of the draw. All in a day's work.

The technicians who perform these jobs must become immune at some level to the emotional distress that many of their patients are experiencing. I don't mean to suggest that I was not treated well anywhere along the way. These jobs involve knowledge and skill, and the practitioners I encountered were professional and competent. But in the end, it seemed not that different from ringing up the groceries or changing the oil. I'm guessing it gets boring.

On that day, I was grateful for the feeling of routine, the technicians' matter-of-fact attitudes. It made me feel less like I was about to die.

Take the first right down the hall. Here's a gown. I'll meet you in the reception area. Are you okay in there? Try not to move. Okay, just a few more minutes. Do you need anything? You're doing great. Okay, all done.

Just another person in line, rather than the tragic case of the day.

On Thursday I fielded calls from the breast cancer coordinator at my local clinic and the patient care coordinator at the breast clinic, both wanting to make sure I knew about support groups, patient resources, help lines, and all the other sources of pinkness available to me. I checked in with Dr. Ryan to make sure he'd heard that Dr. Chen recommended no chemo before surgery, and I let Ashley know that I wanted to go ahead with regular reconstruction with implants, commenced in the same surgery as the mastectomy. Could they all coordinate and get a surgery date on the calendar so we could get this show on the road? Great.

Then I settled in to wait for Monday: the follow-up appointment with Dr. Chen, where I would get the CT and x-ray results and be delivered into the abyss of metastatic cancer, or not.

Chapter Five

I stopped struggling to believe in God a few years before I had cancer.

I had worked at it for quite a while, and I considered myself a "seeker." I went to church, but to a church where it was okay to believe one week and not believe the next week. To go because you believe that God is in the community rather than in the sky. I am a minister's kid, and church *was* our community. I met Jeff in Sunday school, for heaven's sake. I was in eighth grade, the new minister's kid. We were sitting in a circle, on chairs too small for fourteen-year-olds, meant for younger kids. He was the funny kid, wearing high-water brown corduroys, white socks, and brown loafers. It was love at first sight. Over the next couple of years, we played a lot of cards in the youth room during services.

I took the requisite decade off during my twenties, but then returned to church when I had kids, as many seekers do, because I wanted our kids to know the stories and be part of the community. I also believed, and still believe, that searching for ultimate truth is a fundamental part of being human, and going to church is one way to engage in that search. But on Sunday mornings, I sat in a pew near the door, where I could make a quick exit if I needed to.

I also thought that church would provide a posse: like-minded people of various ages who boost each other over life's obstacles. Like cancer. About this, I was not wrong.

But one cold, starry night in winter 2009, we were heading home down the corn corridor, a Brahms symphony still knocking around in my head from earlier in the evening. The surrounding cornfields, tucked in for the winter under blankets of snow, stretched for miles in every direction, reflecting the brilliance of the moon. I looked out the window and thought: I cannot believe there is a higher being who takes a personal interest in any of this.

I also thought: if I've been searching diligently for fifteen years, and I am still not finding, then maybe it's time to stop searching. Maybe that's the answer.

And my search was over, halted somewhere just north of agnostic.

But in 2010, when I suddenly had cancer, and I had to face the real possibility that the end was near, I wondered whether I should rethink my decision. This was the test, perhaps. If falling down, childhood emotional trauma, and bug repellant did not give me cancer, did I have cancer because the Universe Had a Plan for Me? Did I need to believe that God was involved in this personal tragedy, so I could trust there was a reason? Or could I live with the conclusion that it was random? The errant ice cube on the tile floor? The wooden step slippery from the passing shower? The rogue cancer cell no different, really, than the unique snowflake?

This thinking, that Things Happen for a Reason, is common. But I saw no reason in cancer. The idea that cancer happened to me for a reason, because God Intended It, seemed as self-indulgent as the idea that I had cancer because I fell down three times and struck out. My brain wanted such an answer, but that didn't make it true.

So as I faced that Monday appointment, where I would receive either the good news or the bad news about the CT scan, I felt some relief that I'd already decided, before I confronted the impending existential crisis. I didn't have to change my mind. My life, whatever portion remained, was in my own hands. As it always had been. Even if I was going to die sooner rather than later.

I respect others who make the opposite decision: that God *does* have a plan for them. That things, including cancer, *do* happen for a reason. That decision takes as much contemplation and courage as any other. But I don't believe some of us are right and some of us are wrong. I just don't know. Everyone afflicted with cancer has to stitch the experience into the larger fabric of what they believe. Cancer does not just affect our bodies. It gets at the fundamentals of who we are. I didn't want that to be true. I wanted to be unchanged by cancer. But that's not how it works.

Many people afflicted with cancer have made these theological decisions before the crisis hits, and find comfort and strength in their faith, which doesn't budge with cancer. I'm sure that many are also completely thrown by cancer—it shakes their faith, or whatever scheme they have decided on—and on top of the medical gauntlet, they spend a lot of energy struggling mightily with these Big Questions.

And some resist thinking about the Big Questions. Others believe that somehow they can protect people afflicted in their bodies from the consequences that ricochet around in their psyches. It used to be common to not even acknowledge that a person was terminally ill. Sometimes, doctors didn't even tell the patient herself. But my point is, it's a fundamental part of being human to wonder why. To question. To look for the answer. Settled or not, the questions will present themselves during cancer. You have to give yourself space to dwell, and you may have to ask those who love you to respect that space.

• • • • •

Jeff and I saved our marriage in 2008. Sam was graduating from high school, and in a few years, Elena would be out the door as well. So like many couples, we turned around, looked at each other, and said: Do I know you?

A keystone in the architecture of our revitalized relationship was visiting all sixty-seven Minnesota State Parks, which gave us a common goal to work towards. It also gave us lots of time together, driving and hiking, to talk about our relationship problems and answer the quintessential, mundane question: Can This Marriage Be Saved? As a bonus, we could do most of our crying and yelling in the woods, away from the kids. So by 2010, when we needed to have an important conversation, we headed to a state park, by force of habit.

Afton State Park, on the wild and scenic St. Croix River, the boundary between Minnesota and Wisconsin, is one of our favorites. On that Sunday, before. That Monday, the woods were the darker, dustier, crispier green of late summer, when summer has just passed perfect ripeness. The trees had started to dry out a bit, nodding to the inevitability of fall, then winter, although there was plenty of warm weather left. At that point in August, the native growth has given everything it's got for several months, desperate to propagate, to ensure the next generation, in the short time it has. And the tangled mess of vegetation, which has been creeping upward towards the sun all summer, has started to fall down under its own weight and to decay where it falls. The forest floor was abundant, profligate, overwrought. To me, the forest looked cancerous.

We headed up through the browning prairie, where the sun bears down intensely in August, then down the cooler ridge path to the river. From there, the trail runs along the riverbank for several miles. Every time I head down that ridge, I congratulate myself on overcoming my naturally parsimonious nature (minister's kid) and investing in decent hiking boots. Wouldn't want to fall or anything.

We both knew, without saying, that we had gone to this park, where we felt connected to each other and to the earth, to have The Talk. What if we got bad news tomorrow? What if they saw the shadow on the scan and gave me the thumbs down? How would we live out the next six months, twelve months, two years?

Some people might choose to wait. To avoid that conversation until it becomes actually necessary. Until the news is in hand, making you itch and bleed. The dog nose in your face that you cannot ignore. Some might avoid the conversation even then, and never have it at all.

As I followed Jeff down the steep and rocky path towards the river, the pattern of hair on his neck as familiar as my own hand, I dreaded speaking the words. I had no map for this conversation. Maybe, I thought, we should just enjoy these waning days of summer. Maybe I worry too much. Maybe everything will be fine. Maybe this conversation will have been unnecessary.

But I couldn't wait. When I went into that appointment on Monday, I wanted to have a plan. If I was going to die, I wanted to know how I was going to live through it.

I opened my mouth.

So, if we find out I'm going to die, what will we do?

Our feet crunched on the gravel cascading down the path, and I could hear woodpeckers calling to each other across the canopy of trees. Jeff reached back and offered his hand, but we kept walking, stepping over roots and exposed rocks.

If you die, he said, focusing on the trail ahead, I know I will eventually move on. It will be the worst thing that has ever happened to me, and I can hardly think about it. But if we get bad news tomorrow, I want to do everything we can to make the rest of our time together as good as it can be, every day. So how do you want to live the rest of your life?

I dropped his hand and pulled my bandana out of my pocket to dab at my nose, which always drips with exertion.

Well, I'm pretty happy with how we're living our lives now, I said. Doing this. Seeing our friends. Eating great food. I might quit my job sooner rather than later, and there might be some trips I want to take if I feel good enough. But our life is pretty great right now, and I'm pretty happy.

My boot slipped on some loose gravel, and I slid a few inches down the incline. Jeff reached out to catch my elbow. With my bandana, I wiped away a few tears.

My biggest grief, I said, would be not seeing how things turn out for the kids. Although I guess you don't usually get to see how things turn out for your kids in the long term. But I'd like to see them launched and know they will be headed towards reasonably happy adult lives. Maybe I'll make it that far, even if it is metastatic. People can live a long time. My friend Angie lived eight years with stage four ovarian cancer. I'm pretty healthy overall.

I agree. Jeff said. I don't really want anything to change. I know our life will change if the cancer is metastatic. It could be a long haul, and I know it will be hard. But I'd like to keep living like this as long as we can. This is the life I want. I love you, and I think we've done a great job building a life we love together.

We reached the bottom of the ridge, where the path follows an old railroad bed, wide enough to walk side-by-side. Jeff swiped at his eyes, and shooed away a cloud of mosquitos, then took my hand once again. The browning, just-fallen leaves crunched underfoot as we followed the path upriver.

The conversation took only a few minutes, and it didn't get much more complicated than that. We agreed. The plan was this: stay the course. Keep walking. Keep living our life together, until the very last day.

We didn't have to find out if that plan worked. But actually, we follow it even now. Crisis doesn't have to lead you to change course, even while it may sharpen your focus on your current course.

Next to us, the river flowed south, broad and sparkling, on its way to meet the Mississippi. A hawk soared overhead. And the sun arced across the sky, on its way to the next day, and the next.

•   •   •   •   •

We have these ideas about how the world works. That we can ready ourselves for life's perils. That we can keep them at bay by eating right, tending our gardens, and keeping our vices to a minimum. If I play by the rules, I thought, my destiny will be within my control. But despite my compliance, there it was: cancer. I would never be ready for it. The idea that we can be prepared for crisis and the idea that we can keep it at bay are evil twins, luring us into the nether world. For most of my life, I had followed these evil twins down their twisty track.

My desire to have this conversation was, I think, part of my desire to Be Ready, that evil twin. I had wanted to Be Ready for cancer. Now I wanted to Be Ready for death.

I know now that even if you devise a readiness plan, you don't know that it will actually work. Not unlike having babies. You know babies will change your life. You know parenthood will be both difficult and rewarding. But you cannot know, until you are in the midst of it, with that sweet, sweet bundle of flesh pressed up next to you, the exact ways in which it will be hard, or the exact ways in which it will be rewarding. Your murderous rage when the seven-year-old down the block is cruel to your son. Your speechlessness when brilliant prattle emerges from your three-year-old's rosy lips. Your inner turmoil about pushing your teenager to get a job, even though it's not a financial necessity, because getting a job is what adults must do.

I couldn't yet see that readiness was an illusion—an attempt to control the fire hose of life that just keeps knocking you down with experience. And that experience, even when it's out of our control, is the mysterious elixir that makes us who we are.

But I also know that the plan Jeff and I made to stay the course was, and still is, a good one. Evaluating your life, tinkering here and there, or shelling out for the big overhaul, so you are living the way you choose, is worth it. Not because it makes you ready. Not because it makes you safe from the world's hazards. But because it helps you remain present in every moment, so you can make the most of whatever experience comes your way.

•   •   •   •   •

The story of the follow-up appointment with Dr. Chen is short. And Bonnie is the hero.

I slept well the night before, dreaming of over-abundant, past-peak greenery. But in the morning, I could barely breathe as we headed down the highway to the interstate. The overcast, grey sky pressed down upon us. The usually tangy iced tea in my travel cup had no flavor. A few drops of the finest mist fell on our windshield.

Suddenly, lights flashed in the rear mirrors. The county deputies patrol the corn corridor pretty closely, I suppose because it generates easy revenue, and Jeff does tend to have a tiny little tendency to speed on occasion. But he was not speeding that day, ferrying me to my destiny. He was careful and solemn and brilliant, on board with our plan to stay the course. So were these flashing lights another test of my resolve to disbelieve in God? Was the Universe delaying my sentencing, punishing me for my extreme agnosticism? Or was this just Stupid Metaphor Number Three?

Jeff made that noise he makes, which is exactly the same noise his father makes in those situations, swore, and pulled over. The police car pulled in behind us. A young female officer appeared at the window and asked for license and registration. She disappeared back to her car.

We waited. Impatiently.

She reappeared at the window. The reason I stopped you, she said, is you have metastatic cancer, and you are going to die.

No, she did not say that. That's just what I expected to hear.

The reason I stopped you, she said, is it's raining, and you did not have your lights on. Minnesota Statutes Section 169.48 says you have to have your lights on when it's raining. I won't ticket you today, but here's a warning. Please be more careful.

Let me just say: it was not raining. Our windshield had caught, at most, three droplets of mist while we barreled down the highway at fifty-five miles per hour. I think the deputy was brand new, first day on the job, and her colleagues had her out practicing traffic stops for laughable offenses. Maybe even as hazing, not for practical experience. Delaying people with better things to do. Like make it to the oncology office on time for the death sentence.

Was this comic relief? Or perhaps a new basketball game, designed to distract us once again from the gorilla running across the court?

Jeff started the car, and we resumed course. He turned the lights on. I turned up the music and settled in for the drive.

•   •   •   •   •

We arrived at the medical facility on time, despite the nascent deputy, and made our way through the now-familiar maze of hospital corridors to the oncology clinic. We waited with the sad, sick people and doleful cocoa makers, and then were ushered back to an exam room by Bonnie.

Bonnie asked me about my pain level, took my blood pressure, and reviewed my medications. Then she went to fetch Dr. Chen. As she walked towards the door, past my chair, she leaned over and whispered in my ear, clearly against protocol: You're fine. Don't worry.

Jeff started to cry.

It didn't really matter what Dr. Chen said after that, or didn't. My death was not imminent. I had a long road in front of me, but if I turned on my headlights, I'd probably make it to the next county without another traffic stop.

Chapter Six

Maybe I was fooling myself, but I believed I would know if I was meant to die of this disease. Despite my angst-ing before the CT results were in, I had a strong feeling I was not going to die of cancer, at least not in 2010. The Monday appointment just confirmed that I was right. But I might have had the same feeling and been completely wrong. It's just a belief, after all. As I've learned in therapy, not everything you believe is true. (E.g. You're not so special. You have to do this all on your own.)

If you don't count the fall on the slippery steps, my one near death experience occurred in 1988. I was driving east through Minneapolis on Interstate 94, aiming to swing through the University of Minnesota campus to drop Jeff off at school as I headed to Saint Paul for work. Just before Interstate 35 peeled off to the north into the tangle of campus exits, a truck ahead of us ran over a long piece of metal, maybe the arm of a pallet lifter, which had fallen onto the highway. We could see this happening several hundred feet in front of us as we sped into the quantum future.

The metal arm arced into the air in slow motion and began its glacial flight towards our car, like a bullet in a Matrix movie. Tick. Tick. Tick.

Jeff started to scream.

There was no time to react. No time to swerve. I drove right into it.

As far as I could tell, in the ten years that passed in the ensuing split second, that piece of metal was going to come straight through my windshield and decapitate me. Jeff would die in the resulting fiery crash.

But then I knew: I was not meant to die that day.

It tore through the driver's side of my insubstantial Ford Fiesta, like a new can opener through a can of tuna, and left a violent, jagged gash that ran the length of the door. For the next week, before the door was replaced, when we were stopped in the right lane waiting for a light to turn green, the driver in the next car over would roll down the window and shout, what the hell happened?

The window in my door shattered, and I was showered with glass. I pulled over and got out of the car to take a look and brush off the glass. I saw the gaping wound in the side of my vulnerable little Fiesta, and I realized in that moment if I did not get back in the car right then and start to drive—ease into the left lane, move over to the Washington Avenue exit, let Jeff out in front of Coffman Union, head east down University Avenue—I would never get in a car again. So that's what I did.

I recognize the contradiction between my belief that I was not meant to die that day and my rejection of the idea that Things Happen for a Reason. I looked at my children, my life's work, my friendships and joys, and I thought: this is why I did not die in 1988, before any of this existed. How can we survey our legacy on this earth and not think it matters in the larger scheme of things? The physical manifestation of our existence is right in front of us. So substantial. So present. That weight and presence, and our pleasure in it, makes it seem inevitable.

But at the same time, I thought, how can we look at the suffering in the world, in both our own narrow experience and in the overwhelming mass of global experience, and believe that there is intention here?

Did I believe that the good was inevitable, and thus I could take no credit, but the bad was not, and thus I should carry the blame?

To navigate those early days with cancer, I had to keep living with this contradiction. I had to believe that I was not yet meant to die—that there was a larger plan. Otherwise, why suffer through the obstacles looming ahead? Why not give up right away? But I also had to reject the idea that this calamity was happening for a reason. If it was happening for a reason, then I could not control for adversity in my life, and all my compliance had been for nothing. I didn't have time to stop and sort it out. I had to put everything I had into surviving the moment.

So in August 2010, there was no time to swerve. I drove right into it, believing this was not my time to die.

●　　●　　●　　●　　●

My surgery was scheduled for Thursday, August 26, 2010. That was the earliest possible confluence of Dr. Ryan's schedule, Dr. Smith's schedule, and the required six to eight hours in a surgery suite at Abbott Northwestern Hospital. That left me about two weeks with nothing to do. I'd have to go in to see Dr. Smith again to sign some consent forms, and I'd have to schedule a pre-surgical appointment in my home clinic, but those were minor details. I had arranged to take the first six weeks of the semester off, so I did not have to prepare for classes and was essentially off the hook at work.

It's hard to resume normal life under these circumstances. Do you slow down, shed your outer life, divest yourself of responsibility, so you are prepared for the underworld of surgery and chemotherapy? Or do you speed up and cram as much life into those two weeks as possible?

Friends jumped in to ease my way, even in this time when I needed no physical relief. People brought me cookies, calming teas, and chocolate. We went out to dinner and to a Twins game. I received books, crossword puzzles, and trombone music on DVD to help me pass the time. I went for walks and out for drinks on the patio at the Contented Cow, the local pub on the Cannon River. (One evening at the Cow, after overhearing my TMI story about my adventures with the handsome Dr. Smith, which I was relating to a bunch of women friends over a bottle of wine, a complete stranger came over and told me he would pray for me. Embarrassed about over-sharing in public, I blushed to my core and apologized for disturbing his evening.) I hugged Ruby and brushed her yak-like coat. I was shored up and told I need not do this alone. And I started to believe it.

I also became aware of how many tasks in daily life are keyed to the future. My academic semester was scheduled to begin the Monday before my surgery, and we had a new instructor who needed some mentoring before classes began. So I spent a couple of hours with him doing a brain dump: here's what I know about teaching our subject; here's what we're going to do in the spring. I ordered a crate of peaches from the local co-op to put up in the freezer, not knowing if they would arrive before my surgery, or if I would be able to eat them in the spring. I focused on how good they taste in February. I went shopping for new clothes, even though I did not know what my shape would be in a few weeks, because my colleague Angie, who had survived stage four ovarian cancer for eight years, told me before she died that buying new clothes means you believe you're going to live.

I even went to class the first day of the semester. There they were: forty fresh-faced students, eager to begin their journey into law school. I stood in front of them and said, I'm your professor, Mary D. I love teaching, and I look forward to getting to know every one of you. But I have cancer. I'll see you in six weeks. Here is my very capable replacement, Professor Bentz.

I didn't know if this would be the weirdest thing that happened to them that day, or if the first day of law school is so weird anyway, they wouldn't even blink.

Their eyes were on the future. They didn't blink.

•   •   •   •   •

A friend's husband, a doctor, is connected to an Institute for alternative healing affiliated with the hospital where my surgery was scheduled. He recommended that I get in touch with the Institute, which could provide various alternative medicine services for me, both before and after surgery.

I'm open to alternative medicine in most of its forms, as long as it supplements traditional medicine and does not try to squeeze out lifesavers like antibiotics and surgery. But some alternative medicine feels too condemnatory for my taste. If only you get your thinking on track, believe deeply enough, let go of your negativity, you will be healed—it's in your power. I can't get past the blame factor there. Nonetheless, I've tried acupuncture, homeopathy, and herbal supplements, because I believe we don't know everything there is to know about how our bodies and our universe work. Progress is slow. It's not so long ago that we were bleeding each other with leeches and marking the edges of maps with sea serpents. I'll try anything that seems unlikely to harm me.

So I made an intake appointment with a counselor at the Institute and found myself in her office a few days before my surgery. I told her my story, and she told me what services they could provide while I was at the hospital. Music therapy. Aromatherapy. Massage. Acupuncture. Sign me up, I said. She gave me a handout discussing pre-surgery affirmations that I could repeat to myself between now and then, and then she asked me about grief. How was I handling my grief?

The truth was: Not. I think the technical term for it is "stuffing it way down deep into the pit, so you don't have to think about it." I had cried some early on. I had mentioned grief in my conversation in the woods with Jeff. I had cried tears of relief after the CT results. But I hadn't delved into my grief, not the way I needed to.

Grief ripens, until it splits and oozes, like overripe tomatoes forgotten on the kitchen counter, attracting fruit flies and starting to smell. And it is not susceptible to neat packaging. You can't just clean it up and move on. With the tomatoes, I'll get around to chopping them up and slooping them into Ziplock bags before they get too bad. Then I'll throw the bags in the freezer and know they're there, contained, for use in something more complex, a nice pasta sauce for instance, at a later date. Or I'll just throw the tomatoes in the compost and be done with it. Grief just keeps oozing across the countertop.

At this point, my grief was still ripening. Maybe leaving a slight stain on the counter, a little sticky spot, but not yet overwhelming me. I'd felt it split open a little more the previous weekend, when we'd had sex for the last time with my body intact. Otherwise, I had let it sit, ignored but not forgotten. I knew the time would come when I would have to scrape it up and put it in some package, neat or not, and store it away somewhere. But I wasn't ready.

The counselor suggested that I might need to say goodbye to my breasts. I might need a ritual, something to mark this passage. In fact, it strikes me as odd that we don't, for instance, take pictures at these difficult junctures in our lives. We take pictures at other critical junctures in our lives, and we pay big money for just the right scene, just the right lighting. We wouldn't think of getting married or graduating from school without commemorating the event with pictures. Why don't we do that with significant sad moments in our lives, when we will never be the same again? What happened to the tradition of deathbed photography, anyway? The historical society shop in downtown Northfield sells sepia-tinted postcards of Frank James, of James Gang fame, laid out on a wooden board down at the livery barn, bullet hole in his forehead. Shouldn't we mark the occasion when we are about to experience a major loss, so we can remember the before and move into the after? So we can process?

But the thought of saying goodbye to my breasts made me snort, although I kept a straight face in the counselor's presence. What was I going to do? Go around cradling my boobs for three days? Lovingly sing *Bye, Bye Love* or *In the Sweet Hereafter*? Light a candle and burn some sage, pulling the fragrant smoke towards my naked, vulnerable chest?

I don't regret dispensing with a ritual. I know that I was not ready to part with my breasts, and nothing could have helped me be more ready. I had a significant, aggressive cancer. Time was of the essence. I needed to move forward quickly and process the grief later.

When the counselor asked me the question, how are you handling your grief, I did not cry. In fact, I put her off. Fine. I'm fine under this grey sky.

• • • • •

On the day of my surgery, I got up and walked the dog, careful not to eat or drink anything, as instructed. It was a beautiful, mundane August day, with just a little tang of fall in the air. In that last week of August, the mornings start to feel dimmer, and you begin to remember that months of pitch-black six a.m. walks await you, just around the corner. But it's not a bad feeling. Just a reminder of the passage of time.

I put on a sweatshirt and let Ruby take her time as she sniffed out recent neighborhood events and left her doggie Facebook post on the hydrant. We needed to be at the hospital at ten a.m. for the injection of the super-ecto radioactive concoction that would help them map my lymph nodes during surgery. Surgery was scheduled for one o'clock. Despite the clear sky, Jeff promised to turn on the headlights, because you never know what's waiting for you out there on the highway.

We parked in the massive ramp attached to the hospital and decided to leave most of my stuff in the car, where Jeff could retrieve it later, once I had a room. We were early, and we could take our time walking through the ramp, into the building, and down the long corridor to the registration desk.

We trooped down the echoing stairs in the parking ramp, choosing to take a brief detour outside, across the hospital driveway, rather than stay in the skyway. Then we stepped out into the warm August air. There was a little parched grass in the hospital courtyard, and a scrawny tree or two visible across the way. But mostly it was a hard, angled space, where concrete, brick, and asphalt still held the summer heat, all of it grimy with car exhaust and the litter of humanity's comings and goings.

When I stepped through the parking ramp door into that unlovely place, I froze. Maybe it was fear, creeping up from the hard nut that constitutes the deepest part of my brain. Maybe it was actually higher rational thought, suddenly realizing what I was headed for. Maybe the two finally were working together, prodding me to think it through one more time.

I stood among the cigarette butts and gum wrappers, the hospital complex looming around me, blocking the late summer sun, and I thought: I still have a choice. I can turn around now, go back to the car, get in, drive back to Northfield, and take my chances. I do not have to mutilate my body just because They tell me that otherwise I will die. The doctors will shrug their shoulders at this no-show, and someone will probably call to see what happened. They might even try to change my mind. But the cancer police will not come screaming to my door, prepared to wrestle me to the surgery suite against my will. I may survive for years. Some do.

But if I go in that door, twenty feet away across this stretch of asphalt, I will no longer have a choice. I will then be inside, and the wheels of the machine will start to turn. They will take away my clothes, and hook me up to one tube, then another. Then they will put me in a hospital bed, send Jeff away, wheel me down a hall, and park me in a room. They will ask me to count backward from 100, but I'll only get to 95, and then I'll be gone. And when I wake up eight hours later, I will be irrevocably changed.

Until that moment, I hadn't really thought I could choose.

When Sam got really sick with his Crohn's Disease, at about age seventeen, his doctor started talking about taking his colon out. I know it sounds awful, he told Sam, especially at your age. But most of my patients feel so much better once they have the surgery done, they're kicking themselves for not doing it earlier. You are really sick. You don't even remember what normal feels like.

But Sam held firm. He was not ready. He was willing to try the scariest of drugs, drugs that put him at risk for a fatal brain infection, rather than part with his colon at the age of seventeen.

As his mother, I didn't understand. I just wanted him to feel better. To live a normal life, where he did not need to be within sprinting distance of a bathroom at all times. For heaven's sake, Sam. Just get it over with and move on. I didn't push him. But I didn't get it.

In this moment, between the parking ramp and the hospital door, on the asphalt littered with trash, I finally got it. My body was my body. I wanted it intact, even if it meant certain death. A fierce wind blew through me, urging me back to the car.

Don't misunderstand. I was not afraid. But I did not want what was coming. I was not ready to choose. I did not want to choose. Choosing seemed impossible.

But I also did not want to die. What about Paris and Thailand, and Elena's wedding? What about grandchildren, and those last few state parks?

I looked at Jeff, who had stopped beside me and taken my hand, and asked, Is this the right thing to do?

Yes, he said, tightening his grip. This is what you need to do. You need to do this for you, and for me, and for our family.

I swallowed my panic, we crossed the driveway, and Jeff opened the door.

• • • • •

The next few hours were hilarious, in their way, despite the fact that I started crying part way through, leaking ungovernable tears from the corners of my eyes even as I carried on conversations and followed directions. I know that "hilarious" is a strange characterization of my last precious hours with an intact body, when I wasn't ready for this choice and choosing felt so raw. Maybe it's just too painful to think of it any other way. But being back in the company of my dream-team surgeons, trying to say goodbye to my breasts at the same time, was generally an undignified affair. We did not take pictures.

Once we entered the hospital, the ritual commenced, as I knew it would. Registration, followed by waiting. Insertion of tube, injection. Waiting. Separate from Jeff, follow nurse to pre-op cubicle. Strip clothing and bag belongings, recite health history, wait. Jeff reappears, then more waiting, but at least together. Insertion of another tube, more waiting. Consult with anesthesiologist, review medical history again. Meet chief surgical nurse. Wait.

In my experience, the only upside of hospitals is the warm blankets. You can collect a whole pile of these while you wait for whatever comes next. But on this day, I was given the mother of all warm blankets: a giant purple Bear Paws® surgery gown. The gown attached to various hoses, which blew warm air right into my personal cocoon, so I had my own little ecosystem for the next eight hours. This gown far surpassed the Luddite warm blankets. According to the manufacturer's website, Bear Paws gowns are engineered to "clinically pre-warm patients for surgery," which sounds a little, um, alarming, like the microwave just wasn't working that well. But I was quite comfortable, even though I felt like that naughty girl in Willy Wonka who eats too much candy, balloons into a giant blueberry, and floats away.

Once I was settled into my warming cocoon, Dr. Ryan appeared. He interviewed me to make sure I knew what I was there for and that I really meant to be there. Did I? In any case, I signed the paper. Then he asked me to stand and helped me untangle my various in-tubes and out-tubes so I could drop my blueberry suit to my waist. Next, he took out his Sharpie marker and mapped out his plan in some detail. On my chest. Cut here. Stitch here. There be dragons. Then, with a flourish, he signed his name above each breast. See you in surgery.

Just as I was recovering my dignity, Dr. Smith appeared. Once more, we reviewed what I was there for and whether I had the game plan straight. Then I untangled the cords again and dropped the purple gown. He took out *his* Sharpie marker to map out *his* plan, which was even more extensive than Dr. Ryan's plan, so I ended up with basically a map of the London Underground on my chest, Dr. Smith the Circle line and Dr. Ryan the Piccadilly. Dr. Smith signed his name on each side, above Dr. Ryan's name, patted my shoulder, and was gone.

I understand surgery safety protocol. I understand that mistakes get made. The wrong limb is amputated, the healthy kidney is removed, and the diseased one remains. When I'd had Lasik surgery in 2003, I was quite heartened when my eye surgeon drew a large **R** on one cheek, an L on the other, so there would be no confusion during a momentary lapse of concentration. But that was kind of like making up for Halloween. Haha. Isn't it funny to label your face? Maybe it's performance art.

But of all the humiliations of breast cancer, somehow, having two men, basically strangers to me, draw on my chest and then sign their names, like I was a school art project or an electrical wiring diagram sketched out on the sheetrock, was the nadir, the bottom of the deep, dark anaerobic sea. That's when I started to cry.

I had to pull myself together, though, because soon, my alternative medicine pre-surgery practitioner arrived. I don't remember her name, but let's call her Sally. I'm still not clear what qualified Sally for this job, other than a kind and sympathetic nature. At the appointment with the alternative therapies center, I'd said sure, send me everything you've got, because who knows what will help. And I really appreciate the fact that someone out there is trying to make the surgery experience more tolerable, to integrate the emotional with the physical, to attend to the whole, not just the parts. After all, I felt violated because two men had just signed their names on my chest, even though I had consented to them doing so. I needed someone to tend my soul.

But in the end, despite the good intentions, the alternative medicine services provided more comic relief than soul-tending. First, there was the "music therapy." Remember, this was 2010. For at least 5 years, I'd had an iPod, loaded not only with the aforementioned life-saving audiobooks, but ready to play 5,000 of my favorite songs at the touch of a button. The iPod connection was hardwired into my car, and I would have had it hardwired into my brain if that option were available. Jeff had my iPod in his pocket, earbuds snaking into a tangled coil, because I wouldn't risk putting it in the plastic "belongings" bag that would be shipped to my hospital room during surgery.

When I was told that I could have music therapy during surgery, I envisioned Mozart and Shubert piped into the surgery suite for my eight-hour stint of unconsciousness, nourishing my soul while it strove to bear up under the assault on my body. What Sally brought me was a Walkman. With cassette tapes, rattling around untidily in a canvas tote. I thought the Walkman was banned in the U.S. in about 2005, due to extreme anachronism. The one she had in her tote looked a lot like the one I spent way too much money on in 1983, so I could have music on my semester abroad trip to England. I guess they need to fund the alternative therapies program a little more fully.

I declined the music therapy and asked what else she had in her bag of tricks.

Next up: aromatherapy. I have to say I have my doubts about the efficacy of aromatherapy, but as I said, I'm happy to try most anything. Aromatherapy oils, tapped out of their tiny brown apothecary bottles onto snowy cotton balls and stuffed into various air vents, had certainly improved the situation when a mouse built a nest in my Toyota's air filter, lived in it for several seasons, then died. Sally waved several bottles under my nose and asked me which one spoke to me. I chose lavender. She nodded her approval and told me it was calming.

Then came the scientific part. Sally took out a cotton ball, shook a few drops of oil onto it, and pinned it to the left shoulder of my blueberry suit. Now I was a blueberry that smelled like lavender. If you are feeling stressed (!), she said, you can just turn your head and inhale, and the lavender will calm you. Maybe, I thought, we should saturate two cotton balls and shove them up my nose, because I clearly need the maximum dosage.

I turned my head and sniffed. I did not feel calmed. But hey, the cotton ball stayed pinned to my gown for several days. Who can say it didn't help?

The last offering was hand massage. As she worked my muscles and joints, Sally chatted and commented on my long fingers and strong hands (I can't find gloves that fit) while tears dribbled down my cheeks and pooled in my ears. But hand massage was not making me any more ready to face the life-altering knife that awaited me. After a few minutes, Jeff stepped in and said, I think maybe we just need to be alone now. Thanks for everything.

Sally packed up her canvas bag, said a few last kind words, and left. We were alone.

Jeff pulled the privacy curtain shut, then took over Sally's chair by my side and handed me tissues as I cried. The clock on my cubicle wall said 11:43.

I'm sorry, I said. I know it's the right thing to do. I'm just not ready. I keep thinking about waking up and not being me anymore, being some other person with some other body. I didn't want this to happen. I don't know how to make myself feel ready.

My purple suit suddenly inflated with a swoosh of warm air. I dabbed at my eyes.

I know, he said. It's a big unknown. But we will work through this, whatever happens. We're going to have a lot of years to do that. We have a lot of hiking to do and TV to watch. I want you to be with me for that. The kids need you. I need you. Ruby needs you.

He leaned his forehead onto my shoulder so I couldn't see his tears.

The cubicle curtain clattered open, and I was surrounded by movement and green scrubs. I let go of Jeff's hand, and he faded to the background, his role in this scene complete. The orderlies unlocked the wheels on my bed with a jolt and wheeled me through the double doors. I entered the world of bright lights and anonymous faces, concealed behind masks, where you will not remember what happens to you in the next few hours, or what kind of music they play. There was a sudden burst of activity — compression boots on my feet, props under my arms, positioning of my head, checking of tubes. I briefly saw Dr. Ryan, arms bent, gloved hands hovering near his shoulders, just like a TV doctor. Then I counted backward from 100 but only got to 95. And I was gone.

.   .   .   .   .

I awoke to the sound of Dr. Smith's soothing baritone voice, telling me a story. It was a story about how well it had gone, how I was going to be fine. I came around while he was mid-sentence, but I had the sense that he had been sitting in the chair at the end of my bed, long, relaxed legs crossed while he talked, for some time. Talking to me even though it was not clear, I could hear what he said. The clock ticking away on the wall of my cubicle said 6:50 p.m. I had been gone for about seven hours.

I was drugged, incoherent, catheterized, and in pain. But in that moment, I felt alive. The soothing voice continued, lulling me awake, midwifing me back into the world. Dr. Smith stayed with me until I was conscious, and for this, I was extremely grateful. When he patted my foot and left, I knew I would soon be ready to brush off the glass and get back in the car.

Chapter Seven

In 2012-13, Jeff and I rented an apartment in downtown Minneapolis for a year, a temporary escape from small-town life, where the company is good, but the restaurants are dismal. It was a post-cancer indulgence, a seize-the-day moment, a declaration that I was actually going to live, and we should figure out what that meant for our future. In the resulting hiatus of home responsibilities and regular social life, I began to write about cancer.

That spring, a few blocks from our apartment, a teenaged couple from Wisconsin jumped to their deaths in the Mississippi River, off the magnificent Stone Arch Bridge. If not for the HVAC unit on the building next door, I could have seen it happen from my balcony.

It was a beautiful spring night. The moon set in the western sky around midnight, and tree blossoms were just starting to add that fecund scent to the air. The day had been unseasonably warm, and the stones of the bridge would have retained a little heat from the sun, even in pre-dawn hours. I slept through it.

While I have never experienced the despair that must have precipitated this unspeakable tragedy, I do understand the impulse to jump into the river. Many times that year, I stood over the river, in the middle of that same bridge, the powerful current whipping up foam and turbulence beneath me, seeming to flow in a thousand directions at once, and I thought: what would it be like to give myself over to a power so all-consuming? To surrender to the ungovernable forces of nature and let my fate befall me?

I also thought: how can you not want to live to see what happens next?

Choosing treatment is like choosing not to jump into the river. It means you have to keep walking, get to the other side of the bridge, and solve whatever problems were rattling around in your head when you stepped onto the bridge in the first place. You may be tempted to let the powerful current have its way. But I say, keep walking.

•   •   •   •   •

I was transported from post-op to my hospital room around 7:30 p.m. that night. The orderlies wheeled me through different double doors, not the ones that had swallowed me into surgery, down some long halls, into one elevator, up, out, down some more halls, maybe another elevator, until I was wishing they had put some Dramamine in the IV mix. Then I was in a small room filled with bustling people. Someone said one, two, three, lift, I felt a surge of pain, and then I was in a different bed and seemed to be alone.

All sorts of things happen around you, and to you, while you are disappeared into that mysterious land of anesthesia. People play music, have conversations, come and go, cut you open and stitch you back together—and you will never remember any of it. But when you awaken, the evidence remains. Some of it anyway. After a bit, I started to come around enough to mentally inventory my body and assess the damage. My hands felt pinned to my sides.

I started at the top. Head: woozy, and hair undoubtedly a wreck. The least of my worries, of course, but a girl notices these things. Throat: quite sore, hard to swallow. This is what happens when you spend six hours with a tube jammed past your tonsils. Open sore at the left corner of my mouth, presumably where the tube nestled itself in for the duration. Chest: throbbing pain, completely mummified in ace bandages wrapped over gauze. How do they wrap that ace bandage and gauze around and around you when you are on the surgery table? Do the minions hold you up in a sterile embrace while the doctor tosses the gauze over and under, over and under? Do they make jokes about the doctor's pitching skills while they do this? Who supports your head?

Also, the sides of my chest had sprouted tubes, which appeared from somewhere beneath my ribs and terminated in plastic bulbs, not unlike the bulbs you use to clear the snot from a baby's nose, but transparent rather than blue. These were drains, which would collect the red and amber fluid flowing from my wounds for the next several weeks, wreaking havoc with my wardrobe and forcing me to sleep on my back, which I hate.

Moving down. Stomach: ugh. I have never tolerated anesthesia well and felt likely to barf any minute, which might be problematic since I could not sit up. But I could see the golden, kidney-shaped barf-catcher someone had placed nearby, just in case. Arms: an IV snaked up my left arm, which was odd because when I went into surgery, it had been in my right arm. Bruises blooming on my right arm proved it. Must be a story there, but oh well. Bladder: no problem, since I was catheterized for easy, no-fuss service. Legs: confined to the compression devices that inflated with a whoosh every couple of minutes, giving the blood in my lower extremities a boost back up the pipes, in case it was inclined to linger lazily at the end of the line.

Soon, Jeff arrived, bringing my precious iPod and other belongings not entrusted to the plastic bag. He pulled the chair up near the bed and took my hand once again. He smiled.

You look great, he said. I mean it. You do not look like you just had a six-hour surgery and lost some body parts.

I have perennially pink cheeks and a generally healthy aspect, and surgery had, amazingly, not robbed me of it. When I rose from the dead the next day and made my way to the bathroom for the first time, the mirror suggested I'd maybe not had the best night's sleep; but overall, my face was completely normal. I expected pallor, dark circles, bursting blood vessels, ennui. But no, I could have gone to Macy's right then, and the clerk would have looked up at me and asked about my plans for the weekend. Which raised the question, once again: how could this have happened to me when I am clearly so healthy? And yet, how blessed, to be so healthy and ready to rise up and move on.

Jeff settled into the chair at my side, computer on his lap, keys clicking away, and I drifted in and out. It seemed like hours passed, but it couldn't have been long since I hadn't gotten to the room until seven o'clock.

Eventually, I came around enough for us to decide that he should go home and be with Elena instead—another one of those hard choices he had to make. Sam had taken a car and driven with friends to Chicago for the weekend, so he was getting text updates and keeping busy. But Elena had been at home by herself all day, maybe with friends around, maybe not. In any case, she's the kind of girl, especially at that age, who needed a parent to come home and process this hard day with her. Jeff and Elena usually processed together over some Indian food and a nice father-daughter TV show, like *Veronica Mars*. Jeff had been sitting in a bad chair in a soulless hospital waiting room all day, working on his computer, and he could clearly use some Indian food and a few hours vegging out with Elena.

So soon it was me and my iPod in a dark, quiet room, waiting for whatever would happen next.

•   •   •   •   •

Not much happened.

Hospitals are funny that way. Between my own problems and Sam's Crohn's Disease, I spent a lot of time in hospitals for a few years. When Sam was first hospitalized, when he was almost fifteen, it was a total carnival.

Would you like to meet a dog!? No, I'm fifteen, and I have a huge dog, who I don't like very much, at home.

Would you like to make a terrarium!? Uhh—no.

Would you like to sing some songs with Shelly and her magic guitar!? Hmmm—how cute is Shelly?

Would you like to be on hospital TV with Chuckles the Clown!? Excuse me while I turn up the volume on my Terminator movie.

There were times during this year when, confined to a hospital bed, I would have welcomed a therapy dog sniffing at my feet and a little levity with Chuckles, even though laughing may have caused me pain. Hospitals are profoundly boring, and the only relief is TV that will make your brain ooze out your ears. Post-surgery, I was pretty much flat on my back, not able to sit up at all for twenty-four hours, so I could not have seen the TV had I wanted to. But I guess old people in cancer surgery wards, like me, can't tolerate the excitement that pediatric patients can, although I did receive a daily visit from the Bronze Age volunteer pushing the magazine cart.

I lay in the dark through that night, sometimes in, sometimes out. Nurses came to check on my machines and my vitals, but mostly they left me alone. In the middle of the night, I woke up and listened to the quiet. Every few minutes, my compression boots inflated with a whoosh and squeezed my calves several times, giving my blood an extra boost towards my heart. The catheter drained my bladder. IV tubes dripped fluid into my veins, so I didn't even need to reach for the straw cup on my bedside table except to soothe my aching throat. Occasionally, a machine beeped, or a cart wheeled past in the hall. I had nowhere to go and nothing to do.

I did not have Shelly and her guitar, but I started my own music therapy that night, which I believe helped sustain me through the next six months. Music is written to help us process and describe exactly these unspeakable experiences. The grief of choosing the unchoosable. The fear of change and aging. The anxiety about what comes next and whether the fight is worth it. I had listened to a lot of music in my life, but never in the middle of the night after life-altering surgery, thinking about what the music actually meant, letting it salve my wounds.

I'm a classical music fan, so I reached for my iPod and dialed up Samuel Barber's *Adagio for Strings*, which is scored into way too many tragic movies. But it's used for a reason, and for me, it's never turned the corner and become pedestrian, the way Pachelbel's *Canon* did. It captures the grief of being flat on your back, confronting the infinite sky, in a way that I could not express myself.

I listened to the *Adagio* a couple of times, as I would at least several times a day for the next six weeks. Then I listened to a Mahler symphony, full of good German angst and existential despair, and some of the darker Beethoven. A few weeks later, I would begin to mix in Copland's *Appalachian Spring*, that poem of emergence and rebirth, and Mahler's Resurrection Symphony, and the joyous last movement of Beethoven's Ninth. But I wasn't ready for that yet.

It turned out that this was one of those blessings of cancer people like to talk about: time to just lie on my back, listen to music and do nothing else. Time I'd not had since I was a teenager, when I could not really grasp the depths of Barber and Mahler.

And thus, I began to tend my grief and heal.

•   •   •   •   •

The next day, sometime in the dark early morning, Dr. Ryan stopped in, then Dr. Smith. Both took a quick look at my wounds, and Dr. Smith patted my foot on his way out, which became his signature move. But neither had any news on the biopsies sent out after surgery. A nurse came in and commented on what a nice man Dr. Smith is, then Jeff arrived, and the day began.

The goals for the next two days were to get out of bed, start to eat, get off IV pain meds, and get rid of the catheter. If I could accomplish those four things, I could go home on Sunday.

You know how vampires raise themselves up out of coffins—kind of hinge-like? Like they can only bend at the waist, and all other body parts are in rigor mortis? That's how I felt getting out of bed. I used all of my upper body strength to hinge at the waist, lifted through a wall of pain, and was up. But there I was. I was up. I sat in a chair for a minute, then got back into bed and settled into a reasonably upright position. Jeff stuffed pillows around me, refastened my inflatable boots, and pulled his chair close enough to pat my leg occasionally.

Step one accomplished. A sign that life might return to normal.

I worked on the other goals over the course of the day, napping after each new exertion, then carrying on when I woke up again. Jeff remained on pillow-stuffing duty, occasionally going down the hall to get himself another diet Coke or a bag of chips. He made some calls to friends to deliver status reports and kept in touch with the kids. We had not wanted any visitors because I just needed to rest and recover. The morning was relatively peaceful.

About midday, when Jeff was out of the room, I took a deep breath and decided to assess the real damage. Dr. Ryan had told me in my initial appointment that most "ladies" actually feel pretty good when they "look down and see that there is still something there." It's hard to get much of a look down there, ace bandage, gauze, pain, and all. But I pulled the bandage away from my chest, and I saw: he was right.

Where my breasts had been, there were now small mounds, maybe hillocks or knolls, hummocks even. Nowhere near my previous, respectable foothill-sized C cups, but I could see the possibilities. Incisions concealed under steristrips slashed straight across each mound, adding routes to the Underground map still faintly visible on my chest. The holes where the drain tubes exited my body were a bit distressing, but all in all, it was not the end of the world.

Early in the evening, Dr. Ryan appeared in my room and sat down on the corner of my bed. He looked me in the eye, and I could tell it was not going to be good news. I took the earbuds out of my ears and hit pause on my iPod.

He got right to the point.

You had six tumors, he said. Two on the left. Four on the right. The largest was 6.5 centimeters. We knew your cancer was extensive, but we did not know any one of the tumors was this big. We thought during surgery that your lymph nodes were clear, but further biopsy showed that one node on the right, the side with the biggest tumor, had some cancer cells in it. This means you will need chemotherapy. And radiation. Dr. Chen will meet with you in a few weeks to talk about a treatment plan.

My inflatable boots gave a whoosh, pumping blood to my heart. I set my iPod aside and let the earbuds fall in a tangle.

What could have caused this? I asked.

Maybe a virus, he said. He looked away.

He asked if I had questions. I did. I wanted to know why this happened—biologically, medically, theologically, environmentally. I wanted to know if I would be alive in five years. I wanted to know if chemo is as bad as I feared. I wanted to know whether I should quit my job and live like I had no time to spare.

But none of these seemed like fair questions in the moment. The surgeon is not a research scientist, an oncologist, a priest, or an environmentalist. Surgeons have a job to do, an important one, and they do it as best they can, then move on. I would need to look elsewhere for answers. So I said no, I would follow up with Dr. Chen, and thanks for keeping me informed. Dr. Ryan soon left the room because there really was no more information to deliver. As his steps echoed down the hall, I stared at the wall, not sure how to tackle all these questions at once.

Dr. Ryan handed me into the care of Dr. Smith, because who needs two surgeons once the offending body parts are gone and the bad news is delivered, and I haven't seen him since. At least I got to keep the one who's easy on the eyes.

I lay in my darkened room that night, Jeff home with Elena for more vindaloo and *Veronica Mars*, me playing the Barber *Adagio* on my iPod. I hadn't been ready for this news, any more than I'd been ready for the surgery. But at least I had all the pieces now. I had a lot of cancer, and it was going to be a long haul.

Keep walking, I told myself. Don't look down into the turbulence.

•   •   •   •   •

You know how those Internet ads appear on the right side of your search results screen?

SHOCKING!! Acai Berry Diet!!!! Weight loss secrets exposed!!!

Or

SHOCKING!! 46" 3D LED TV for $84.95!!!

Or

The SHOCKING TRUTH about car insurance prices!!!!

Let's get this straight. Shocking is having an undiagnosed 6.5 centimeter tumor, one of six tumors, which puts you well into Stage III breast cancer, removed seven months after a clear mammogram. Six-and-a-half centimeters is the size of a standard, large-size political campaign button. If I had pinned my HOPE AND CHANGE button to the right side of my chest, it would have just about covered the largest tumor, if only I'd known where to pin it.

As my friend Jackie said later, looking sideways at Jeff over a martini, you'd think SOMEBODY would have felt that.

Chapter Eight

I went home on Sunday, as expected, having attained all my goals. My goal-attaining skills actually tripped me up in this whole cancer thing. Generally, I expect that if you set a goal, exert yourself in the right direction, and work diligently, you will achieve your heart's desire. That's always worked for me. You need to set realistic goals, of course. But if you do, you will be rewarded with success. I viewed living a long, healthy, cancer-free life as an attainable goal, like graduating with honors from college. You eat right, exercise, don't smoke, get your checkups. Follow the rules. Bam. Goal achieved. But I was wrong.

My sister Ann had returned to help run the ship while I recovered. When Jeff and I arrived home, she and Elena got me settled on the brown sofa that would become my parking spot for the next several months, through recovery and chemo. The dog, Ruby, immediately came over and put her nose in my face. Not to be outdone, her sibling rival, Scout, the tuxedo cat who weighs seventeen pounds, jumped onto my flattened chest and kneaded her paws directly on my incisions, because she is an evil genius, the way cats are. Boo, the little white cat, skittered under the sofa, where she stayed for approximately four months. Digby, the cool cat, supervised from the back of the other sofa.

Life resumed around me, and I looked on. I felt like a sizeable rock, parked in the middle of the room, obstructing traffic until everyone adapted to the new traffic pattern. Every once in a while, someone would come sit by me, or on me (e.g. Scout), but otherwise, the flow parted around me and continued on its way while I waved feebly at the backs of the departing figures.

This is not to say my family was inattentive. On the contrary, your family has to figure out just how many times they can ask what you need before you threaten to rise zombie-like from the sofa and punch them weakly in the face. At that point, you don't really need much other than rest and water. So there's not much they can do once they adjust the pillows, make sure your water glass is within reach, and shoo the cat away one more time.

In fact, this absence of need, the want of anything to be done for you, is a potential emotional train wreck that comes with cancer. The people who love you want desperately to make it better. They would do anything to ease your way, even the tiniest bit. This was abundantly clear to me throughout my months of treatment. I tear up even now, just thinking about it.

But the fact is, they can't take it away from you, and they can't go through it for you, and they can't, at a physical level, make it much better. All they can do is sit with you and grieve with you and invite you to be as irrational as you need to be about this stupid thing happening to you.

Some people in your life will understand this: that they can offer nothing more, no matter how much they want to. They do what they can and accept that the little things—sending you a card or a pointless gift, watching dumb TV with you, bringing you food you cannot eat, stopping by for five minutes to check in—add up to "making it better." But some struggle, because they are loving, capable people who can usually arrange things to their own satisfaction, and no matter how hard they try, they just can't pull you single-handedly out of cancer. Watching you suffer and feeling helpless just about kills them.

As the person with cancer, you have to let them be their own crazy selves, just like you have to be your own crazy self, and accept that their anxiety about their limited ability to help shows how much they love you. You may find yourself letting people do things for you that don't really need doing because you hope it will make *them* feel better. And you may find yourself getting cranky that they can't see what you really need, which may be nothing at all. It's a balancing act, like any uncharted territory in life, and everyone involved needs time to figure out how to stay on the tightrope and avoid plunging to the hard ground below. My advice: assume everyone around you is doing their best, and let them love you. You would do the same for them.

During this time, I had to continue to resist my inclination to go it alone, to argue that I didn't need help. I did need help. Lots of it. Accepting the sweet affection and care that so many people poured over me didn't cure my cancer or lessen my physical pain or keep me from barfing. But sharing the same space, even momentarily, with people who loved me made even this otherwise miserable period totally worth living.

Like it or not, that's a lesson learned.

•   •   •   •   •

Sunday evening, I rose from the brown sofa and took a walk around the block, Ann at one elbow, Jeff at the other. Summer had turned into fall during my stay in the hospital, and while it was still warm, leaves crunched under our feet, and the light was fading early. We chatted with neighbors, including Carolyn, who got worried about the slightly mottled blue hue of my hands and called her retired physician father to get his opinion. But my hands are always that color, probably because all the blood is in my healthy pink cheeks, and the walk was otherwise uneventful. I got home and checked "walk around the block" off my goal list.

Bedtime at home that first night involved a new, strangely intimate ritual that I had to get used to over the next several days. The ritual was called Stripping the Drains.

After a mastectomy, you have these tubes sprouting from somewhere inside your chest, exiting through small, open holes in your skin, snaking around the front, and ending in the aforementioned squeezable bulbs. You pin the bulbs to your "supportive undergarment" so they are not hanging around your knees, knocking about uncomfortably and fighting gravity. Before you shower, when you are allowed to take off your supportive undergarment for twenty minutes, you have to dig out the lanyard from the last conference you went to and pin the bulbs to that for support. Otherwise, they pull uncomfortably at the exit wounds in your sides, making you wonder what body parts they might bring along if they suddenly pop out.

The "supportive undergarment" is really just a sports bra that zips in the front. You have to wear this for six weeks after surgery, day and night, partly so you have something to pin your drains to. And partly, I guess, so everything stays put where the doctor stitched it. And you have to call it a "supportive undergarment" so the doctor knows you are a serious person and don't think this is a joke. Following Dr. Smith's instructions, I drove forty miles to the breast cancer accessories store (Guess what? It's all pink!) in a distant suburb to purchase my supportive undergarments, at a highly inflated price, only to find that I could have bought basically the same thing at Target. It would have been called a sports bra and cost about one-third as much. But hey, Blue Cross was paying, because that's one of the perks of breast cancer: your insurance company has to pay for your bras. Who knew?

The whole drain scheme is a brilliantly engineered, natural vacuum system that slowly sucks wound fluid out of you, so you don't puff up, fester, and burst. The drain's bulbs have little caps that snap on and off so you can squeeze the fluid out into plastic specimen cups, measure it, and contemplate just how disgusting our bodies really are before you pour it in the toilet and flush. The goal is to exude under ten ccs of fluid per day from each drain. The reward for achieving this goal is having the drains removed so you can sleep on your side again, as God intended you to.

The drains also create a temporary wardrobe crisis, especially when you have purged all your oversized clothes in an effort to lose the frumpy. Not that there's anywhere to go during these couple of weeks after surgery, or any way to look in this condition but frumpy. But still.

In these first post-surgery days, I could neither find my armpits nor raise my arms. The surgeon digs around in there, getting the lymph nodes out, and that whole underarm area takes issue with that. So I was pretty swollen and misshapen. And when I tried to lift my arms to lower a window and shut out the autumnal evening breeze, I could only get them about half way up. So much for reaching above the stove for the salt.

So there were some tasks I very much needed help with, including stripping the drains.

Basically, to strip the drains, you hold your left thumb and forefinger at the top of the tube where it exits your body so that you anchor the tube and it does not pull on the exit wound. Next, you take an alcohol wipe between your right thumb and forefinger, so you have a little bit of lubrication but not too much, and you pinch the wipe around the tube and slide your fingers down. As you slide your fingers down the tube, all the fluid and clots, which may or may not resemble small mammals, that have collected in the tube over the course of several hours move down the tube and into the collection bulb at the end. You take several passes down the tube this way until you're sure it's cleared, then you squeeze the bounty into a specimen cup for measuring. Finally, you write down the time and the amount on the drain-stripping schedule form they gave you at the hospital, so when you go back to see the surgeon, you can verify that you've been compliant.

I'm sure there is a fancy scientific name for this bodily fluid, but I never learned it. And, although I don't like to admit that I noticed, it's a surprisingly beautiful color. As I healed, the color changed from a rich, ruby red, not unlike the velvet of a Christmas party dress, to the deep amber of an October hardwood forest. If the color were captured in stained glass rather than in a bodily secretion, you would hang it in the window and hope the light hit it just so in the morning. Over several weeks, it becomes paler and paler, like a jilted Victorian heroine, until the doctor pulls the tubes from your chest. After that, it disappears into your body, joining all the other secret and beautiful processes hidden within, instead of wending its way down the drains.

Ann and Jeff divvied up drain-stripping duty over those couple of weeks, but Jeff volunteered for the first round, that first night home. I sat in the dim light of the bedroom on the edge of the bed, looking away while he collected cotton balls, alcohol wipes, and the towel to catch any mess. Pictures of my children and unread books cluttered the bookshelf next to the bed. The dog lay on the other side of the room, panting, doing what she could to keep me safe.

I wished this was not happening, that I could just curl up on my side and go to sleep. How could I allow another adult, for whom this was not a professional obligation rewarded with a decent salary, to perform this extraordinarily intimate and disgusting task?

You don't have to do this, I said. I can do it. Really, I can. Give me the wipe.

I lifted an arm and held out a hand. My hand shook, and pain radiated down my side.

Jeff didn't look up. Shut up, he said. I mean that in a nice way.

Hold, pinch, slide. The fluid moved down the tube and into the cup.

Jeff held the cup up to the light and squinted at the numbers on the side. The dark red fluid glowed.

Ten CCs, Jeff said. Good job.

He headed into the bathroom. I heard the tinkle of fluid being dumped into the toilet, then the flush. I lay back on the bed and shut my eyes.

Between them, Jeff and Ann repeated this ritual dozens of times over the next several weeks. Each time, I protested. No, I can do it myself. Each time, they said some version of, Shut Up.

Gradually, I moved a little closer to accepting that this was an act of love that showed just how deeply they cared about me.

•   •   •   •   •

The second day at home was busy. Not for me, because my only job was to lie rock-like on the sofa, petting the dog (or the cat) for exercise, to the extent I could move my arms. But the crate of peaches had arrived, the farm share was delivered, a friend's daughter showed up because she needed a bed for a few nights before she started college, and Sam returned from Chicago.

Ann organized the kids to slice and freeze the peaches, to sort and store the farm share, and to cut the last of the summer sweet corn off the cob and squirrel it away for the winter. She tidied, got groceries, did laundry, and arranged the many flowers delivered to our door. Elena's friends came and went because it was the last week of summer and their senior year of high school started next week, so they had important hapless loitering to tend to. Jeff had work to do, so he sat in the chair near my sofa, poking away at his computer, ready to drop everything and do my bidding if I had a need.

In other words, it was very normal, which was my preference. Because life goes on, and the future beckons.

Over the next few days, we established a routine. In the morning, I got up and, with Jeff or Ann, we stripped the drains. Then I went downstairs, maybe ate some yogurt or toast, and lay on the sofa while Ann and Jeff did the morning chores. Next, Ann and I walked around the block, at which point I'd be ready for a little nap. After my nap, Elena emerged from her room and Sam came home from his morning work shift at the library, so we chatted while Ann made some lunch. Then we went upstairs, where Ann stripped the drains so I could lie down and listen to *Adagio for Strings*, or maybe some Copland as the week wore on. Ann is a psychologist, and at the time, was expanding her practice into meditation and alternative therapies, so she downloaded a guided meditation podcast, which I listened to before falling asleep again.

When I woke up again, dinner would either be delivered by friends or in the making. In the meantime, someone walked the dog and cleaned up the cat pee, took a head count for dinner, and set the table. My job was to lie on the sofa until dinner was on the table, sit up for the thirty minutes it took us to eat, then return to the sofa for a little TV before more drain stripping, then bed.

It is hard to let go of everything around you when you are usually captain of the ship. I had at least thirty years of domestic supervisory experience behind me — washing dishes, mopping up the floor, handing a child the carrot peeler with a maternal "get to work," folding the towels, running to the store for bean sprouts, wiping down the countertops — and the voice from those years whispered in my ear that I'd better get busy or everything was going to fall apart. Because how could it go on without me?

You are in this terrible position, where you want to know it can go on without you because it must. But at the same time, you wonder what it means that it *does* go on without you. If you die of this horrible disease, will you not be missed? Will your family adapt, recalibrate, so the ship will sail ahead unimpeded?

In fact, the ship will continue to sail. Not that you won't be missed. You will be. But none of us is indispensable. The most important and most beloved people who have ever lived, whoever they were, have died, and the world has moved on. It is human nature to adapt and adjust, despite our losses and attendant grief. So you have to come to terms with the facts: your family needs you while you are alive, and they will always love you. But if you die, although they will miss you terribly, they will move on. Because that's how life works.

In some nebulous way, of course, I'd known this before. We are mortal. We die, and the world barely blinks. But before, I had always imagined that it would happen when my usefulness was at an end and no one depended on me or looked to me for anything, after I'd spent years winding down, once I'd gotten used to the idea. Granny's been in her rocker in the corner for days. Has anyone checked to see if she's alive?

But I have now seen that life goes on without me. And that's both a terrible and wonderful thing.

•   •   •   •   •

For the next few nights, at bedtime, after the drain stripping ritual, I would shut myself in the bathroom and pull the supportive undergarment and ace bandage away from my chest and look at the wreck of my body. The signatures and London tube routes had washed away, and I was beginning to look less bruised and swollen. I had this fixed idea that I looked like Gumby, minus the green, of course. I no longer had contours and recesses, but seemed somehow two-dimensional. A flat rhomboid, wider at the top and narrower at the bottom, with arms sticking straight out the sides. No armpits. Bending my Gumby arms gingerly, I would splash water on my face and neck and lather up with my grapefruit-scented organic face wash. After patting dry, I would slather on the cool, white, anti-aging night cream that I'd been using for years to stave off wrinkles.

Then I would look in the mirror and wonder: what's the point?

Chapter Nine

If you are supporting a person living with cancer, you may wonder whether anything you do makes a difference. You can't take the cancer away. Often, you can't make your loved one more comfortable. Sometimes, they may not even register that you are present, or may be unable to acknowledge your care. As a support person, you may begin to doubt that your efforts are worth it.

With cancer, you have to accept that you can't fix it. That's the reality. But doing something, one thing, whatever it is, matters more than you might realize. That became particularly clear to me during this time—post surgery, pre-chemo. Even the smallest gestures made a difference, although I couldn't always respond in the moment. And together, the multitude of small gestures wove a net of care that, in the darkest hours, kept me aloft.

The gifts, offerings, and messages I received humble and sustain me to this day. It was a mountain of generosity, an ocean of kindness, more than I can ever give back. Every day brought a reminder that I had a team, a cheering section that wanted me to reach the treatment finish line. And, even more, wanted me to live well and feel loved while I ran the race, no matter what the outcome.

Food had begun to arrive shortly after my diagnosis. Chocolate chip cookies, still warm from the oven, appeared on the front porch. Blueberry muffins arrived, moist and sugary, on a paper plate, and homemade jam and bread, in a basket with fall apples and golden raspberries. An out-of-state friend who shares my cake obsession even arranged for her mother to drive two hours to deliver a cake from a locally renowned bakery.

After my surgery, for months, friends and neighbors brought full meals to feed my family. A childhood friend brought the biggest pan of Minnesota goulash hot dish I had ever seen. (Macaroni noodles, ground beef, and tomatoes, all topped with cheese and baked for an hour—ultimate comfort food. Delicious.) It would have fed us for weeks.

Although meals arrived at planned times, when we actually needed them, we couldn't eat it all. Only Jeff, Elena, and I were home, and I was not always up to eating much. It was thousands more calories than we could consume. Some nights, I sent my family around the neighborhood with the extras, looking for someone who needed dinner tomorrow or would appreciate half a cake.

Besides food, there were cards wishing me well, offering prayers, sharing a few heartening or humorous thoughts. Cards from friends and colleagues, friends of friends, friends of family, family of friends, the guy who mows my mother's lawn. Flowers and plants crowded the living room, giving even our cats a smorgasbord to snack on. People called just to check on me and chat. They prayed for me for months.

Then there were tangible gifts—gifts for comfort and consolation. Three prayer shawls, an afghan, and a quilt, all hand-made. A microwavable, aromatherapy teddy bear. Silly things and serious things, angels and mugs and inspirational pins. Every gift was designed to buoy me, in the most comfort possible, from one miserable day to the next.

There were also less tangible gifts. People offered to drive me places, clean my bathrooms, walk the dog. A few days after my first chemo, a colleague organized "Hi Mary" day at work. She made a sign that said "Hi Mary" in a dozen languages, took pictures of colleagues holding the sign, and emailed them to me one by one during the day. The pictures flooded my inbox, about sixty pictures in all. Every picture made me cry. Even now, when I edge back towards cancer gloom, wondering why this happened to me, I pull these pictures up on my screen, and each face lifts my spirits.

One golden September day, just before I started chemo, my book group friends brought lunch to share on my patio. That summer, my family had moved into a new house, and the surrounding landscape was barren. So along with lunch, my friends brought plants dug from their own gardens. After we ate in the warm fall sunshine, the dog crowding our feet under the table, catching both the shade and the stray food scraps, they planted the hosta and ferns and daylilies, then watered the garden from the rain barrel. I looked on from my chair, grateful to be reminded that spring would come next year, certain that I would be here to enjoy it.

Our friends were generous and followed their hearts. Now was not the time to worry about waste or waistlines, or whether I believed in prayer or not. This abundance, this feast, was about so much more than the calories we required to get through the week. Every card, every last drop of salad dressing, was a gift that helped us cope, a message that we were embraced and cared for.

I may not believe in God. But I believe that this abundant generosity, this community embrace of a person in need, is as close to the divine as we get. Even if food is not necessary, or cards go unopened, or gifts have no palpable purpose, small efforts fill the room with reminders of why we are here. Although I know that surgery and chemo and radiation saved my life, I am certain that this generosity accounts for my actual survival. Despite my grief and pain, and my fear of what would happen next, the expressions of love that came my way, piece-by-piece, word-by-word, made it a rich time to be alive.

• • • • •

About ten days after my surgery, despite all the outpourings of love and support, my grief tomato began to rot in earnest.

My sister Ann went home, and the visiting college student moved into the dorm. Sam packed up, kissed me on the head, and moved his stuff to campus. Over the weekend, Elena and her friends made their annual trek to the Renaissance Festival, which left the house quiet, foreshadowing Tuesday, when school would begin. Jeff wouldn't let me walk Ruby yet, lest she injure my still-healing arms with her sled-dog momentum. But I was up and about, walking more, and off pain meds. And I was reaching my limits with lying on the couch. From that vantage point, I found myself cataloging the dust bunnies under the furniture and contemplating the grime on the windows. So I figured I must be healing.

On Monday, I had a walking date with a friend. So I got up and began the routine: strip the drains, eat my toast, carefully insert my arms into the sleeves of an oversized shirt. But somewhere in the process, I began to split open.

Something in me let loose. I started crying, and I could not stop.

The first month of cancer—the diagnosis, the medical spanking machine, the juggling of logistics so life can go on without you for the weeks after surgery—takes everything you have to give. During that time, you focus on making the necessary arrangements and screwing up the necessary courage to choose to live, whatever it takes. Like deciding to have the baby, then decorating the nursery. You don't have much time to think about what comes next, but you know it requires new curtains.

Then there's the surgery and its aftermath, when you are in pain or on meds or still foggy from the anesthesia. You don't have a lot of processing power, and what you do have diverts to the physical realities of healing.

But on that Monday, Labor Day, ten days after surgery, the new normal began to settle in. My body had healed enough that I could begin to function like a real person, even strip my own drains. At the same time, the practical plan for the next month required nothing of me. Before I started chemo, my only job was to continue to heal and regain my strength. So on that day, I emerged from hibernation, took stock, and thought: what the hell?

During the moment of paralysis in the hospital driveway, I could not indulge in an hours-long crying jag while I agonized about what I was doing and whether it was the right choice. Instead, I locked down my grief long enough to get to the surgery suite, where they sent me into blissful oblivion until the deed was done. But the lockdown was over. The hatch opened, and the river began to flow.

I lay on the bed, wanting only to curl up on my side in a fetal position and sob. The unfairness of having unmanageable drains sprouting from my sides, which made a fetal position physically impossible, only made me cry harder.

I moved to the bedroom floor, where, huddled in the corner by the bed, I could become as fetal as possible. Jeff came to check on me, and he sank to the floor next to me when he saw what was happening. It's okay, he said, putting his arms around me. It's okay.

Between sobs, I managed to choke out a few words, asking him to call my friend and cancel my walk. He left the room long enough to make the call and to talk to the kids, because their mother was sobbing audibly in the bedroom, and to accept the food that someone delivered to the door. Then he came back, grabbed the tissues from the dresser, and settled in next to me on the floor for however long it would take.

It's okay, he said again, pulling me closer, even though I resisted. It will pass. You're going to be okay. Whatever happens, you're going to be okay.

He held on tight. He smoothed my doomed hair. He didn't let go.

It was hard to believe in that hour that I was going to be okay. I was inconsolable, incoherent, completely turned inward. I was furious that this was happening to me and terrified of not seeing how the story ended, of dying too soon. This was not in my plan. I thought I had done everything I could to prevent it from happening, and yet here I was. How could I continue to live in the universe where this happens? I was stranded in the midst of this dark, implacable storm, Wagnerian and tumultuous, and I didn't know how to escape.

I continued to sob, oblivious to the world outside my dark corner, outside that room, outside that house.

A few summers before, on a warm August morning, one of those freakish but increasingly common super-storms passed through our town. Thunder roared and lightning flashed, and hail the size of grapefruits punched holes in windows, playground equipment, and lawn furniture. People carried injured ducks into the veterinarian's office, hoping she could save these creatures that had been stoned nearly to death by Mother Nature. During the storm, I was on the highway, driving north to the cities, and it was as if I'd been dropped into the middle of a baseball game played by giants throwing Olympic fastballs.

I lacked the imagination to understand that I should pull over, preferably under a bridge, because one of those hailstones could come right through the window and knock me on the head. Luckily, the hail didn't breach my windshield—which was merely cracked and shattered—but it did go through many car windows in town, leaving violent, jagged holes that tempted exploration with a fist. Every roof within a five-mile radius was ruined.

But that day, although it left devastation in its wake, the Wagnerian storm passed, and people emerged to clean up the mess. The ducks were buried. The deck chairs and plastic kiddie pools went in the dumpster and were trucked to the landfill. The windows and roofs were replaced. Every once in a while, years later, you might still pull in next to one of those hail-damaged cars in a parking lot. But most of them ended up flattened at the salvage yard.

And so it was. My storm passed, as these things do. I can't account for the time that morning, but eventually, my sobs wound down, and I accepted a tissue and a glass of water from Jeff. In the corner, I leaned into him and told him I didn't want to die, but I would try to be brave, whatever happened. He held me close and told me he would be there no matter what, a message I needed to hear over and over during this time.

And after a while, I took a deep breath and got up to bury the ducks and reset the patio furniture. I washed my face, went downstairs, and told my wide-eyed children that I was grieving, and I didn't know how long it would take. But I was still here, and that's what mattered. Then I lay down on the sofa and let them turn on dumb TV and sit with me while I pivoted back to the life ahead.

•   •   •   •   •

As I write this story, I'm aware of how many times Jeff held my hand or passed me tissues or patted my shoulder, how many hours he spent next to me in his chair, computer on his lap, tending to his external responsibilities, but ready to reach out and pull me up, physically or emotionally—whatever I needed in the moment. That stormy Labor Day was one of the more memorable moments.

You may wonder, did Jeff ever let me down during this cancer experience? Did I ever reach out my hand, through the tangled vines of the cancerland jungle, and come up empty?

I have to tell you. Looking back now, my answer still has to be No.

It's not that Jeff has never let me down. We've had as imperfect a marriage as any other couple still married after thirty-odd years. We had years and years of me not asking for enough and then resenting that I didn't get it, and him working too hard because it felt better than grappling with the stuff of emotions.

But a couple of years before I had cancer, we worked together with a brilliant therapist who taught us the skills to stay connected, no matter what. To get over ourselves and offer that hand, no matter what. And, amazingly, those skills worked. It was almost as if getting through cancer together was the dissertation crowning our Ph.D. in relationship skills. Cancer gave us the opportunity to practice, over and over, what we learned, and we just kept getting better at it.

Looking back now, I believe that most significantly, Jeff never made *my* work harder by asking me to bear his grief about my cancer. I'm sure I checked in with him about how he was feeling, and I'm sure his friends and colleagues did too. I know he talked to friends about it when they asked. When we talk about it now, he tells me he felt grief and fear, and anxiety besides, about what his life would be like if I died and he had to move on. I may joke about him taking up with the cute forty-something around the corner, but it wouldn't be that way. He would grieve, and he would miss me the rest of his life. But he dealt with it mostly internally. So he was always able to show up for me with a positive attitude and practical assistance.

So, yes. My bull, born in the year of the ox, was a solid brick wall of stability during this time. It's true that he likes to sit in his chair in our living room, and maybe move to his chair on the porch during fine weather. But he was also happy to sit in the chair next to my hospital bed or in the chair in any number of endless medical waiting rooms, even though, at the same time, his sixteen-employee software company—his "hobby," not his real job—was going through a major business reorganization. There have been plenty of times in my life when his inclination to sit in his chair with his computer on his lap has made me crazy. But this rock was exactly what I needed to cling to during cancer.

Over many months, Jeff rose periodically from his chair to clean up after me and take up the household slack and communicate with friends and family and fetch me some water. And best of all, even when I had drains filled with disgusting fluids hanging out both sides of my chest, and when I had lost every hair on my body, he kept telling me he loved me and I was the most beautiful woman in the world.

I chose to believe him. He's a very convincing guy.

Chapter Ten

Then there was the fact of living with cancer. During this post-surgery period, when you are preparing for chemo, you definitely have cancer. You know it. Everyone around you knows it. You are in cancerland, and there is no pretending otherwise. People ask how you're doing, and you tell them the how the surgery went and how many chemo sessions are scheduled. So there is something to talk about, and that's a relief. There are rules for this game, and people generally know them.

But cancerland is all jungle, and you're fighting a war in that jungle, and the perspective from within gets a little distorted. For instance, you suddenly realize just how much cancer there is everywhere around you. If it's not Celia on *Weeds*, it's Christina on *Parenthood* or Izzy on *Grey's Anatomy*. Not to mention *The Big C*, an entire show about cancer, not just a seasonal side plot, and *Breaking Bad*. There's the horror of pink ribbon month (does that look like a noose to anyone else?), pink coffee cups, and pink garbage trucks. Really. Can we please just stop talking about cancer?

I found new reasons to pick fights with the people around me, who were only trying to help. Poor Jeff, doing the laundry a few weeks after my surgery, caught hell when he put Elena's bras in my clean laundry pile. Hadn't he noticed that I had no breasts? That those cute, lacy bras, candy-striped and beribboned, could not possibly be mine, and never would be again, imprisoned as I was in the supportive undergarment and drain apparatus? On bad days, I resented plants sent to the house because they were something more to take care of when I could hardly take care of myself. Then there were male friends and colleagues. During conversations, their eyes would flicker to my chest to assess the damage. Please don't pity me, guys. I can be a real woman without my breasts. I would bite my tongue and turn away, knowing that I was entitled to my feelings, but also that their curiosity was natural. A brief social encounter is no time to confront our irrational cultural obsession with breasts.

I found more general targets as well. As part of our Sunday morning hiking routine, Jeff and I sought out the best breakfast in Minnesota. For a while, we were regulars at Barney's in Faribault, chowing down on pancakes and hash browns with the pre-church crowd. But when I had cancer, I suddenly couldn't stand the feel-good aphorisms on the walls, each one painted in careful, fourth-grade cursive above a silk and straw flower swag.

In the end, it's not the years in the life, it's the life in the years.
It's nice to be important, but it's more important to be nice.
Never get so busy making a living that you forget to make a life.
Our glory is not in never falling, but in always getting up after we fall.
Life is not measured by the number of breaths we take, but by the moments that take our breath away.

These saccharine ditties enraged me. There is something both brilliantly trite and obviously true about them, and the weird parallelism appealed to my literary brain, despite the banality. But maybe during this time I was living too close to the bone. Maybe wrestling daily with questions about my actual mortality left no room for clichés or philosophical corn. It seemed we went to Barney's for breakfast just so I could build up a good head of rancorous steam that would bleed into the rest of the day, fueling my forward momentum. Maybe my rage helped vanquish the cancer cells, or maybe I just needed to rage at the world, and stupid sayings painted on the wall were a pretty safe target.

Despite these ups and downs, life crept closer and closer towards normal. I went back to yoga twice a week, even though Dr. Smith told me to wait six weeks. Not so compliant, but I had to rebel *sometime*. I walked a lot, including downtown, to hang out at the annual Defeat of Jesse James Days, where the bank raid that done in the James Gang is re-enacted every hour all weekend, complete with horses and gunshots and dead Swedes, and you can buy cookies shaped like feet—aka De Feet of Jesse James. Get it? You can also eat every possible fried food, preferably on a stick, then ride the Tilt-a-Whirl and throw up. I avoided that part because I knew my immediate future held plenty of barfing. But these were exactly the normal life distractions I needed while waiting for chemo.

In fact, after a few weeks, I felt so normal, when people showed up at our back door with food on Sundays, Tuesdays, and Thursdays at six p.m.-ish, I felt compelled to stop whatever normal activity I was doing and lie down on the sofa under an afghan, so I could feel like I deserved the attention. Many nights during this time, we did not "need" someone to deliver dinner. I was okay; I could have made dinner. I had to remind myself that dinner delivery was about taking care of us, our friends tending to the community, taking us in. But in this stretch of normal, accepting help was especially difficult for me. I said "Yes" anyway. Yes, and thank you.

Because I felt so normal, on the third Sunday in September, a little over three weeks after my surgery, Jeff and I decided to take a more ambitious hiking day trip. We had built our excursions up over the last several Sundays—from the immediate post-surgery walk around the block to a gingerly mile hike on flat ground the following week to a normal-ish walk through the woods the third week. I thought I was ready for something more challenging. So on a late September Saturday, we headed south towards three unexplored state parks: Lake Louise, Forestville-Mystery Cave, and John A. Latsch. The day was warm and brilliant, the leaves at their peak of color, but not yet releasing their hold. The corn still stood in the fields but had turned from green to dusty gold. As harvest approached, the stalks shrank in their rows, like aging soldiers, revealing the rich brown Midwestern soil beneath.

Lake Louise was pleasant and flat, and we had an easy walk by the Upper Iowa River, where a fox scurried across a wooden bridge, its tail a bushy red and white flag flashing in the sunshine. At Forestville-Mystery Cave, we skipped the cave because the day was too glorious to waste it underground—winter would be here soon enough—and instead ate our lunch next to the bucolic Root River, then wandered around the park's deserted historical town-site and autumnal period-authentic garden. Only a few migrating geese and chattering squirrels disturbed the quiet. We stopped in the postcard-perfect bluff town of Lanesboro for ice cream, then wound through the Root River valley towards the Mississippi.

I hadn't done my homework on John A. Latsch State Park, the final stop on our tour. The guidebook said it had one mile of trail, which sounded like a perfect end to the day. But I had neglected to read the fine print. The mile of trail went straight up. For about 5,000 steps. Four hundred and fifty feet up, to be exact. Which is about the equivalent of a forty-five-story building, or the length of Noah's Ark.

This was perhaps Stupid Metaphor Number Four, and I hadn't seen it coming.

We started the climb on the theory that we would go a little way and just see. We could always turn around. So we started to climb. We climbed, and we climbed. The steps seemed never-ending.

About halfway up, panting, my calves aching, I clutched at a tree branch over-hanging the steps.

I don't know if I can do it, I said, leaning over to catch my breath. It's still a long way up.

Jeff backtracked a few steps and landed next to me. I was pleased to see that he was also winded. Maybe it wasn't just about cancer. Maybe this was actually hard.

Okay, he said. We'll just stay here a few minutes so you can catch your breath. We don't have to go all the way to the top.

We sat down on the steps and watched through the trees as a flock of Canada geese honked their way south. The afternoon air was just starting to catch an evening chill in the shade, but the steps were warm and dry. After a few minutes, my heart slowed and my calves relaxed. I looked up the steps and couldn't see the top. Then I looked down the steps and couldn't see the bottom. I'd come this far. Surely I could keep going.

We're pretty far, right? I asked.

Oh, yeah, Jeff said. It can't be too much farther. And the view will be fabulous. Want to give it a try? We can stop as much as you need to.

He stood up and offered me his hand. I pulled myself up, and we began to climb again. We climbed some more, then stopped again, then climbed some more. Jeff stayed in the lead, and I kept my focus on his broad shoulders, which stayed steady, a few steps ahead of me.

And of course, it was not unlike cancer, if you want to think metaphorically. The climb was really hard, and I had to stop to rest a lot, and my doctors probably would have advised against it, and I swore a lot along the way, although I did not cry. But I kept climbing, because what are you going to do? Turn around, without ever seeing the view? Never know what's at the top? So we climbed some more, and I did not burst open or fall down the steps or keel over and die, even though I felt like I might.

We came up over the last couple of steps to the top, then scrambled onto the flat, rocky outcrop that was the highest point for miles around. We stretched up into the sunshine on our aching legs and surveyed the view. And it was indeed awe-inspiring.

The Mississippi, widened by Lake Pepin at that point, stretched out for miles and miles, north and south, flowing through the vibrant fall landscape, which was lush and fertile, green and gold and red and blue all at once. Eagles soared overhead, because eagles always soar over that stretch of the Mississippi, and white sails dotted the water below. We could almost touch the cottony clouds. After a few minutes, another hiker joined us at the top and offered to take our picture. I resisted telling him that actually, I had cancer and was lucky to have made it up the bluff. But here I was. Jeff handed him the camera.

I took in the view and the fall sunshine and the clear air, and I thought: I'm not particularly strong. I'm not particularly ambitious or courageous. But if I can climb this bluff three weeks after a bilateral mastectomy, I can do anything.

Maybe, I started to see, things don't Happen for a Reason. But you find the reason anyway.

Chapter Eleven

My return to normal during this time was punctuated by more doctor visits—surgery follow-up and chemo preparation. About two weeks after surgery, Dr. Smith removed the drains: one, two, three—shlooop, and they were out. I had barely registered my relief before we moved into the "expansion" period of reconstruction, which is an entirely new adventure. Kind of like Westward Expansion from the American History textbook. Onward and outward, to conquer more territory. But on your chest.

Expansion works like this. During reconstruction surgery, the surgeon inserts these tough little balloons equipped with magnetic valves in your chest. Several weeks after surgery, after the drains are out, you put on your sunbonnet for the Expansion Journey, and you ride down to the plastic surgeon's office. There, the doctor uses a magnet to locate the valve, then sticks a needle through your skin and into the valve. He pumps saline into the balloon through the needle, something like fifty ccs a week. Gradually, you expand. Voila. New breasts.

After a mastectomy, the nerves in the chest area are permanently offline, and you never regain feeling there, which leaves you feeling vulnerable and somewhat sad about your sex life. So during the expansion process, you don't feel the needle in your skin. Dr. Smith cut into me for all sorts of reasons after my mastectomy, and I felt it, inexplicably, only in my left collarbone. Usually, he shot in some Novocain, just in case, but I don't see that it mattered. After being cut or punctured with no anesthesia, my body did seem to know some assault had occurred, so it sent out little chemical messengers on little chemical messenger bicycles to alert the system that something distressing was going on. So I'd end up feeling a little "shock-y" afterward, until the chemicals all put their bicycles away. But I did not feel pain.

Each step in this expansion process is called getting a "fill." You go into the plastic surgeon's office every week for a fill, for some number of weeks, until you are again the size specified in your original instruction booklet, unless you are ambitious and want to be bigger, which, presumably, the plastic surgeon will happily accommodate.

If you came of age in the 1960s and 70s, this might trigger memories of Growing Up Skipper. Growing Up Skipper was one version of Barbie's younger sister, Skipper. I have no idea where Mattel came up with the name Skipper. I have never met a real live female person named Skipper. Apparently, I don't hang out with the right crowd. But then, there was no yacht club within two hundred miles of my hometown.

Anyway, Growing Up Skipper was supposed to be about twelve or thirteen, and her beige plastic body was extruded from the Barbie-making machine accordingly. Meaning, she had starter breast bumps, but not Barbie's triangulate Tetons. Growing Up Skipper also had a clever built-in mechanism so that when you cranked her arm, her breasts expanded, because young girls all over America were sitting at home wishing for a doll with expanding breasts. Skipper never quite reached Barbie proportions, but she gave it a good try.

As an aside, Barbie also had a friend named Francie. In endowment terms, Francie was somewhere between Skipper and Barbie. She was a doll made for girls destined to be disappointed with life. Francie's boyfriend was named Allen, and he was not quite as muscular or as shiny as Ken. Francie had no chance with Ken, I expect, because of her obvious inadequacies when compared to Barbie.

The parallels between getting "a fill" and cranking the arm of Growing Up Skipper are inescapable. Both are pretty creepy ideas that I wish I didn't know about. Both rankle at my feminist convictions that we over-emphasize breasts in our culture and breast size doesn't matter. Even as a ten-year-old, I scorned Growing Up Skipper.

But I had committed to reconstruction six weeks earlier, before my surgery, and this was no time to re-examine my decision. So for weeks, I trundled off to the plastic surgeon's office for my fill. In a few weeks, I achieved Francie size, which, like the Francie of my childhood, was not quite satisfactory. Then I held my breath as I approached Barbie-like proportions. After about eight weeks, I was "done." Full Barbie achieved.

Of course, getting a fill did not restore feeling in my chest. But it was a relief to pull a sweater over my head and admire my restored shape in the mirror. And once I was done with the supportive undergarment,

I could go without a bra and no one would know the difference. A minor consolation.

Besides going in for a weekly fill, I started physical therapy three times a week so I could again shut the windows and reach the salt. I went for a post-surgical check-up with Dr. Chen to prepare for chemo. I attended "chemo class," where I watched a video with perky patter and healthy-looking actors discussing the horrors about to commence while affirming that a person could still function normally during chemo. This run of appointments actually helped me feel like I was being productive, not just a lump on the sofa. I was in the business of having cancer, and it took most of my time. But I was on board to do whatever it took.

.   .   .   .   .

The week before I started chemo, I was scheduled for a minor surgery to install a chemo port into my chest, so the poison could be pumped directly into my main blood vessels. The day before this surgery, I saw my primary care doctor—the doctor who delivered the bad news back in July—to make sure I was up to surgery. I had climbed the John A. Latsch State Park bluff the Sunday before—what other proof did we need?—but protocol must be followed.

At the clinic, the young nurse who had failed to return my call back in July settled me into an exam room. She avoided my eyes as she took my vitals and reviewed my medications, then left me to sit shivering in yet another hospital gown while I waited. At least this gown was blue and white, not pink, like so many breast center gowns so far. I was already sick of pink, and I hadn't even started chemo.

The door opened, and my doctor entered, clutching my chart to her chest. She looked me in the eye as she shook my hand. Then she sat down, swiveling towards the desk on her stool.

Well, she said, looking at my chart, I cannot believe what's happened to you since July. I don't know how that January mammogram could have missed cancer that extensive. I looked at your post-surgical biopsy report, and I just couldn't believe it.

Well, I said. Yeah.

I had no script for this situation, so I laughed a little. But I wondered, did someone miss something here? Is that what she's telling me? Should I be thinking about suing someone?

I asked the radiologist to go back and look at the January films, she said, swiveling towards me with her stethoscope in hand, but he didn't come up with anything. Nobody wants to be the interesting case of the week, but you certainly win that prize around here.

I laughed again. But in my head, I imagined the whispered exchanges, the white coats hunched over my chart: six tumors, can you believe it? How did *that* happen?

Yeah, well, I said, you take your consolation where you can find it.

Could those tumors have been there in January? I asked. Could that much cancer have grown in six months?

She swiveled back to the desk and looked down at my file in front of her. We can't really say, she said. On the films, you have very dense tissue. It can be hard to see anything through tissue that dense.

She stood, grabbed the exam light from the wall, and shined it into my eyes.

As she listened to my heart and looked into my ears, I thought about whether I wanted to sue someone. I'm a lawyer, so I'm not afraid of lawsuits. But I also know what lawsuits mean. Usually, in terms of time and energy and addressing harm, nobody wins. Everyone suffers. It can go on for years. And to what end? I had good insurance that was covering the cost of treatment. Suing would not take my cancer away, but it might consume whatever life I had left. Even if I was fine, a lawsuit would sap my energy, impede my forward momentum.

No, I didn't want to sue someone.

The doctor finished the brief exam, typed some notes into the computer, then told me I could get dressed.

Other than this, you're very healthy, she said as she moved towards the door. I'm not supposed to say this, but I think you are going to be fine. Hang in there.

She shook my hand again, and the door clicked shut behind her. The paper on the exam table crackled as I slid my feet to the floor, then I pulled off the latest blue and white gown, balled it up, and tossed it in yet another exam room corner.

As I dressed, I wondered once again how this had happened to me, the queen of compliance. What sequence of actions, then reactions, then misdirected cell divisions, brought me to that room? In those first few months, it was still easy to spiral into wanting to assign blame. Was it my failure to wash my vegetables adequately? Was it forty years of plastic milk jugs and aluminum can linings? Was it my unresolved self-esteem issues? But as I paraded back through the clinic, acutely aware that I was the interesting case of the week, feeling as if eyes followed me as I passed the central staffing desk, I concluded once again that there was no one to blame.

Over the months and then years since my diagnosis, I have had to reach this conclusion any number of times. I have needed to give up my need to know why, my desire to pin responsibility on someone, anyone, even my reprobate self. My doctor didn't know why. My surgeon didn't know why. Maybe science could figure out why, but that wouldn't help much after the fact. I like to think I have made peace with the mystery. None of us knows why, because we live in a beautiful, glorious world beyond our own understanding.

· · · · ·

The next day, I went in to have the chemo port installed in my chest.

You install cable TV or art exhibits or new toilets. You should not "install" objects into bodies. Like the pre-mastectomy map and signatures on my chest, the word suggested I was a technical problem to be solved rather than a person with feelings. As it turned out, the port installation involved some technical difficulties and seemed akin to a weekend plumber installing a sink from Ikea. So maybe install is the right term.

Jeff's classes had started, and the surgery was scheduled for a teaching day, so he relented when I begged him to go to work and let a friend deliver me to the hospital for this minor procedure. At the hospital, I put on another blue and white gown, then got settled into one of the giant blue vinyl recliners they use in same-day surgery prep cubicles and chemo wards. They pad these chairs with blankets to make them less cold and slippery. But as you slide into the chair, you know that the vinyl is insurance against leaking bodily fluids, and yours are likely to be the next contribution. I took some deep breaths and tried to relax.

A nurse appeared and tucked me into the warm blankets. She chatted and fetched enough pillows to put me at ease. Then an IV technician arrived to get me ready for the drip. The cubicle curtain made the familiar whoosh as she pulled it shut behind her, and the resulting current of air cooled my face. The IV tech sat down on the wheeled stool and rolled it close, then leaned in to examine my arms.

Which arm? She asked, pressing a finger into the crook of my right elbow to test a vein.

It doesn't matter, I said. They can both be cranky about IVs—some days more than others.

Let's try the right, she said.

I've never been squeamish about needles, so I watched as she punctured the skin and tried for a vein in the soft crease of skin. The needle moved under my skin like a fish skimming the surface of the water. But the vein refused to be caught. After several minutes, she pulled the needle out and tried another site, with no better success. She tried one in my hand, but there too the vein escaped the needle.

Okay, she said. Maybe we'll have better luck on the other side.

She switched to my left arm, flicked her finger at a promising vein, and tried again. But again, no luck. Each time she tried a new site, I winced as she poked the needle through the skin, then I watched as it moved beneath the surface and I willed the blood to flow. The warm blankets were starting to cool, and I started to shiver. A collection of bruises now peppered my arms. As the tech poked at yet another spot, I looked away from my arm and studied the emergency protocol poster on the wall next to my recliner.

I'm sorry, the tech said, pulling the needle out yet again. I don't usually have to poke so many times. Let's get you some more blankets.

She rolled across the room and pulled opened the curtain. The nurse appeared with more warm blankets and tucked me in tighter. In the hall, gurneys rumbled past and machines beeped and clanged. The IV tech rolled her stool back towards me, leaned in again, and tried another vein.

I'm sorry, she said again after a few more minutes. I'm going to get someone else to help with this.

She went off in search of the nurse anesthetist, the cubicle curtain billowing behind her as she left. In a few minutes, the nurse anesthetist arrived and planted herself on the rolling stool. She examined my arms, then tried to insert the IV into several untried veins—back of right hand, right wrist, back of left hand—all without success.

Wow, she said. Your veins really aren't cooperating today. I'm not sure what to try next.

She went off in search of the anesthesiologist himself. I pulled the blankets up to my chin and shut my eyes. I envisioned lying in the soothing dimness of the yoga studio. Maybe relaxing would help.

A few minutes later, the anesthesiologist pushed the cubicle curtain open with a clatter and marched into the cubicle.

I hear we're having some trouble with our IV, he said. He sat down on the stool, rolled in my direction, and pulled my arm out straight. He sighed as he picked up an IV needle.

I don't know why the nurses can't handle this, he said. I'm already behind schedule. This part is their job, not mine. Hold the arm straight. Don't move. This will just take a minute.

He poked the needle hard into my skin and fished for a vein. I winced, then watched as the vein slid away. He moved the needle this way and that under the skin, but again it refused to cooperate. He harrumphed.

They've already ruined this site, he said. Let's try the other arm.

He repeated the process on the other side, sighing as he worked. I began to believe that my veins' lack of cooperation was a personal failing that could be remedied if I could just muster some moral fiber. I shut my eyes again and returned to the yoga studio, but as the poking and complaining continued, I shrank further under my blankets.

As I watched the doctor move from site to site, switching from one arm to the other, I began to wonder. Was my terror of chemo constricting my veins, making eventual delivery impossible? Was this what they call bodily wisdom—my body's own protest against allowing itself to be poisoned? Because if they could not start an IV, and I could not get a port, then I could not get chemo in a few days. What would that mean? But wait, I thought, I don't really believe in that mind-body stuff, do I?

And where was my lavender cotton ball when I needed it?

The anesthesiologist rolled himself away from my blue recliner and dropped his equipment on a metal tray with a clatter. He stood up. The nurses hovered.

Let's move her into surgery, he said. We're already behind. Wrap the arms in warm blankets and make sure she's hydrated. We'll figure something out when we get in there.

He stomped out.

The nurses scuttled around, adjusting my position and piling on more warm blankets until my actual shape was completely obscured under the mountain of white. They wrapped my arms, helped me drink a glass of water, and gave me a little blue pill to help me relax. Then an orderly appeared to wheel me into the surgery suite. I began to wonder if they would perform the surgery without an IV, to keep the doctors on schedule. At what point should I throw off my mountain of blankets and run?

The surgery suite was cold and bright. I shut my eyes against the lights and tried to feel the heated yoga studio floor beneath me and to summon the non-melodic, new age music my teacher favored. Meanwhile, the epic battle continued: Anesthesiology Guy v. Mary's veins. Who had the requisite moral fiber? The pokes became more insistent, and I gave up wincing. In my head, I switched from the yoga studio to the bluff-top view of the Mississippi the week before. I thought about the softness of Ruby's ears, and Elena's visceral warmth when she curled up next to me on the sofa. I thought about Sam's courage in facing so many needles and scopes at such a young age. I decided if I made it through this procedure, which had seemed so routine when I arrived that morning, I would have my friend take me to the bakery on the way home, where I would get the biggest cowboy cookie they had. Maybe two.

Just as the anesthesiologist was starting to poke needles between my toes, as if I were an advanced stage heroin addict, someone slipped an IV in my arm and a vein caught, as if none of the past thirty minutes had happened. I expected balloons and confetti, but none appeared. The anesthesiologist harrumphed and moved towards my head. Get the surgeon, he said. And soon the welcome, warm fog of anesthesia settled over me.

The port installation was uneventful after that, although I was in a strange half-aware twilight throughout the procedure. A blue surgical drape covered my head (apparently, for the surgeon, it's better not to see the face above the jugular vein you're cutting into), so my brain put me into a dream-like alien world where everything was some shade of blue. I wound through a maze of blue tunnels that sometimes opened into the golf game the anesthesiologist and the surgeon chatted about as they worked—the greens now blue, the sky a paler blue complement—and sometimes into houses I had lived in since childhood, the rooms distorted into freakish blue shapes. As the surgeon inserted the tube into my vein, there was some pulling and tugging that felt oddly mechanical, like extracting a stuck valve from its housing, but not painful. Maybe I was a blue machine, not a body? I thought. The conversation about the golf game continued through the tugging.

And then I was done. Installation complete. Open the gallery doors and let in the crowd.

The orderly wheeled me back to my cubicle and settled me into the vinyl recliner, where I could swim up from the blue anesthetic stupor. Gurneys rumbled past as I struggled to pull myself back into reality, and the bright lights made stars appear behind my eyelids.

As I came around, my original nurse was tucking warm blankets around my legs and my chest. I opened my eyes and looked at her.

Thanks, I said. That feels good.

How are you feeling? Any nausea? She asked. She turned to the wall to dim the lights.

Okay. Not ready to get up yet, but no nausea, I said. I'd just like to sit here with the blankets for a while.

She was quiet for a moment as she returned to fussing with my blankets. Then she said, I've been doing this for a long time. When you've been doing this for a long time, you can tell who's going to make it and who's not. You're going to make it. I have no doubt. I know you've had a tough morning, but you're going to be okay.

She gave my blankets one more tuck, leaned in to hug me, and left the room.

Maybe she says this to everyone. But every patient is hungry to hear these words. It doesn't matter if they are true. Through the wooziness, I registered her kindness in offering them and held it close as I pulled myself together for one more trip home.

A chemo port is about the size of a quarter. It sits just below your right collarbone, like a misplaced Girl Scout badge for Extraordinary Courage. All I have to show for it now is a faint scar, about an inch long, below my collarbone, and another small round scar just above. When I meet new people, I find myself looking towards their right collarbones to see if I can glimpse a scar, so I know if we're in the same club. If our scars indeed match, we could launch the secret handshake, if only we had one.

•   •   •   •   •

Then there was hair. Because chemo, at least for breast cancer, must involve attention to hair. Wig or scarves? Hats are an option, but are they just pretentious? You need to decide in advance and be prepared. If your hair starts falling out by the handful and you don't have a plan, or at least a scarf handy—well, you will definitely not get your Girl Scout badge for that one. For me, anyway, having a plan kept the chaos at bay.

These days, there is a head-freezing device available, so if you wear the freezing cap during chemo, your hair follicles do not react, and your hair does not fall out. I understand that for some women, keeping their hair is akin to keeping their dignity. So the extra expense—many thousands of dollars over the course of treatment, at least in 2010—is worth it to them. I find myself being rather judgmental about this option, even more so than plastic surgery. Hair is a renewable resource—it comes right back for free, starting about six weeks after your last chemo. But breasts do not regenerate. Plastic surgery is your only option, other than stuffing your bra with tissues. So I could justify plastic surgery, but I could not justify the expense of the hair freezer.

In any case, I've had short hair since I cut off my long tresses in a dramatic gesture when I was fifteen, the same week I got my braces off. So where hair was concerned, I figured I'd be back to Go in no time once chemo was over. But I decided to shave my head before chemo so I would not have to deal with losing it in chunks later. I set up an appointment with Samantha and recruited Carolyn to go along for moral support.

I made the appointment for the end of the day at Samantha's salon, so we could have a glass of wine if we wanted and no one would see me cry. I remembered the last time we had to put down a pet, because our ancient, decrepit cat could no longer move from under the bed to the litter box. When we made the vet appointment, they scheduled us for the last appointment of the day. That way, we could sit in the vet's office and sob for as long as we needed to, or at least until our guilt about keeping the vet from his dinner outpaced our grief. The same principle was at work here.

I walked the six blocks downtown with Carolyn, shuffling through the fall leaves, Carolyn carrying the wine and the corkscrew. The salon was quiet, as we had planned, the smell of perm chemicals and shampoo still lingering in the air. I settled into Samantha's chair, where she billowed the black cape around me. It settled around my shoulders with a sigh. Carolyn retrieved some paper cups from the water cooler and poured the wine. We toasted with the paper cups and took a drink.

How short? Samantha asked, fingering my hair speculatively.

Shave it. Shave it all off, I said. I'm ready to get this next stage underway. And I don't want to wake up one morning and find it all over my pillow.

Well, she said, examining me in the mirror as she began to massage my shoulders. How about just really short? Then you can feel normal, more or less, for a few more days.

What is normal? I thought. Is normal still possible? Am I hurrying the abnormal, hoping to move this process along faster? Should I just slow down and see what happens?

Yes, Carolyn agreed. I vote for normal for as long as possible.

And at that moment, Jeff and Sam opened the salon's glass door, bringing the fresh fall air in with them.

This must be where the party is, Sam said. They walked to Samantha's cubicle and leaned in together to kiss my head. I started to cry.

Samantha looked at Sam and Jeff. Really short or shave it? She asked.

Really short, they agreed. Normal for a few more days is good.

Jeff, Sam, and Carolyn stood in a circle around me, sipping wine from paper cups, as Samantha got out the scissors and started to cut. As the hair fell onto the black cape in wet clumps and Norah Jones sang her heart out in the background, I dried my tears and reminded myself that every normal day is a gift.

Chapter Twelve

The chemo leg of the breast cancer journey has a completely different character than the surgery leg. Maybe one is a leg and one is an arm.

Unlike chemotherapy, surgery makes emotional sense. You have a tumor, or tumors as the case may be, and the nice surgeon goes in and takes the tumor out. They send the tumor to the lab, then they tell you all about how big it was and what kind of food it feasted on and how aggressive it was. And you think: the Beast has been vanquished. The white knight went into the cave, fought the good fight, and came out victorious, dragging the dragon behind him for dissection and disposal.

But then you move on to the next part of the story, the less heroic part, where the knight's lesser colleagues go in and hose down the cave, to make sure all the dragon poop is gone. Because, it turns out, the dragon poop can kill you as much as the dragon. And dragon poop is so toxic that you can't hose the cave down with water. You have to use toxic chemicals that threaten to bring the cave down around you, like spraying carbolic acid on limestone walls.

Enough with the cave and the poop. But you see my point. Killing the dragon makes complete sense, but then what? Cancer researchers agree that chemotherapy kills the few errant cells that may have escaped the tumor and may be floating around your body, eager to latch on again given the opportunity. But just how much chemotherapy improves your chances is not clear. If you're a non-medical person, you can read medical articles on this topic until your eyes cross and still be a little unsure whether it's worth it, especially once the chemo starts to take a toll on your body.

Plus, unlike surgery, where you submit, and then it's over, and you heal and move on, with chemo, you submit and then it gets worse. Then you submit again, and it gets even worse. And you have to keep submitting, six times in my case. Each time I wondered whether it was worth it. Each time, at some point, I found myself staring over the edge of the bridge, wondering what would happen if I dove into the raging river and let the current envelop me. I would probably drown, but who knows? Currents can be funny that way.

•   •   •   •   •

Chocolate, white cake, and red grapefruit dish soap. These are a few of my favorite things, which chemo ruined for me, at least temporarily.

Chemo messes with your natural chemical make-up in unpredictable ways. My natural chemical make-up predisposes me to like chocolate. A lot. Preferably dark chocolate, but milk chocolate will do. At least a little bit every day. My grandmother had a special candy dish, manufactured in Pennsylvania by Westmoreland glass, not far from Hershey, the chocolate capital of the world, that was always filled with M&Ms. My mother had the same dish. And I have the same dish, given to me by my grandmother as a wedding present. I had to stop filling it with M&Ms in 2007, or risk arrest by the Weight Watchers police. But in 2010, I was in the habit of eating a few small squares of organic chocolate every night after dinner, just that little something to tide me over until frozen yogurt time.

Once I started chemo, I could not stand the taste of chocolate. It tasted bitter on my tongue, and I found the texture sticky and unpleasant. But I could hardly complain. I was fighting for my life, after all, and children were starving in Africa. So what if I'd lost my taste for chocolate? But still, I believe that life is about the small pleasures, and having this one taken away dented my morale, even more than losing my hair.

As for the demise of my cake monkey, this involved a self-inflicted misstep. My chemotherapy began when cupcake shops were just becoming the rage. A new cupcake shop had opened about a mile from the oncology clinic, and on my first day of chemo, Jeff went out midday to check it out. We were looking for ways to brighten the day, which started badly, and give me a last treat before the hammer fell.

Do not eat anything you love, and would like to continue to love, within a day of receiving chemo. You probably will regret eating anything at all, and when your brain inevitably draws an association between whatever you ate that day and the nausea and vomiting that follows chemo, it will put you off that food, possibly for years. I'm surprised that no one has developed a food aversion therapy involving chemo to help with weight loss. I did not enjoy my birthday cake for the next two years.

And then there was the grapefruit dish soap. I'm generally not brand loyal, but there's this grapefruit dish soap that I really like. It's the least expensive brand per ounce, and it has a tangy grapefruit scent, not too sweet. But Adriamycin, one of the three chemotherapy drugs I received, is exactly the same color: a rich, citrusy red. After my first chemo infusion, my brain decided that any rich, citrusy red substance was a deadly toxin and I should get as far away from it as possible. For several months, I could not even go near the kitchen sink without feeling nauseous because I knew the grapefruit dish soap lived beneath. Looking under the sink and catching a glimpse of the bottle could actually induce me to vomit.

Eventually, I saw reason and accepted that this aversion did not signal a weak character, and I did not need to tough it out. I let Jeff buy lemon dish soap instead, even though the grapefruit bottle was not empty yet. He also moved the grapefruit dish soap to the basement, out of sight and out of mind, because he is a reasonable human being.

Here we are, several years later, and I can again enjoy chocolate and cupcakes, and I think there is grapefruit dish soap under my sink, but I'm not sure, which is a good sign. You don't know, though, when you start chemo, what the little things will be. The things that will stretch your endurance for no good reason and make you consider giving up the fight. You need a big bucket of faith that this too shall pass, as my father used to say. And you have to dip into that bucket regularly for sustenance.

•   •   •   •   •

The week I started chemotherapy was Patient Appreciation Week at my clinic.

I suppose even oncology clinics have competition and need to bring in business to stay afloat. But I think Patient Appreciation Week goes a little too far. What's the message here? Hey! We're really glad you're here! Thanks for having cancer! Please don't die—we need your business!

This is not, of course, the message they want to convey. But still. I suppose I shouldn't fault them for trying to make patients feel good and for brightening up the waiting room a bit, where the atmosphere ranges across the many shades of miserable to grim. But appreciating the patronage of cancer patients seems like dicey territory.

During Patient Appreciation Week, the waiting room had a carnival-like atmosphere. Colorful banners and balloons decked the walls, and trays of cookies and snacks sat throughout the room. When I signed in for my appointment, the receptionist handed me a swag bag. It contained:

A Shane Co. (jewelers) hat

A *Cure* magazine

Two sample-sized tubes of Aquaphor ointment

A key ring from Polar Chevrolet

A coupon for one free cookie from a local bakery

A coupon for one free six-inch sandwich from a local sub shop (some restrictions apply)

A complimentary two-week membership at a gym

One free lane of bowling at Drkula's 32 Lanes (shoes included)

An Edible Arrangements discount coupon

A Minnesota Oncology brochure

Two miscellaneous zippered pouches, both emblazoned with drug company logos

Oh, twenty-first-century marketing.

On that first day of chemo, I was having a bad day before I even arrived at the clinic. Earlier that morning, the surgical steristrips covering my incisions for a month had given up the last threads of adhesive and wilted off my chest in the shower. As I looked down through the steam and rivulets of water and examined my incisions for the first time, I realized it wasn't a pretty sight. The wounds were crusty, red, and inflamed. The right-side incision had several wide scabby spots, where the skin did not quite meet in the middle, and pearly white connective tissue peaked through the gap. I washed my hair quickly and tried not to look down.

When I got out of the shower, I carefully patted myself dry, then covered the angry incisions with ointment and gauze. I armed myself in my supportive undergarment, pulled on my chemo pants, the comfortable sweat pants I had bought just for the occasion, and topped it off with a soft, loose-fitting shirt that provided easy access to my port. Then we set out, Jeff driving, lights on, to Dr. Smith's office for my fill, the first stop of our day.

Because the first chemo loomed in front of us for the day, we had an early appointment at Dr. Smith's office. The office was quiet, and Jeff barely had time to reach for his computer before Ashley appeared to usher us back to an exam room. As we settled into the room, she handed me the usual pink tissue bolero jacket and told me Dr. Smith would be right in.

I hadn't seen Dr. Smith himself in a few weeks because Ashley had done the fills once my drains were removed. So this was our first encounter since the full pathology report came back—the one evaluating my six tumors, giving them grades and scores, like scholarship recipients. Although Dr. Ryan had delivered the basic tumor news the day after my surgery, I was nervous, unsure whether the news could get worse now that the full report was in. Jeff moved his chair closer and put his arm around me as I shivered.

Dr. Smith swept into the room, Ashley close behind, and offered his hand to me and to Jeff. As I got comfortable on the exam table, Ashley set to work opening the sterile tray containing the fill equipment while Dr. Smith pulled on exam gloves with a snap. Then, pushing my bolero jacket aside, he moved the magnet across my chest to align the fill valves and pumped in another fifty ccs on each side. He handed the equipment tray over to Ashley with a clatter, told me I could sit up, and sat down to look me in the eye.

Because your cancer was more extensive than we thought, he said, reconstruction is going to be more complicated. Radiation, which you need to have on your right side because of the extent of the cancer, and reconstruction don't mix very well. The irradiated tissue shrinks and loses its pliability. We don't generally do reconstruction this way when radiation is involved. But we're on the road now, and we'll just have to see how it goes. After we finish the expansion process in a few weeks, we can't do anything more until four to six months after radiation. We can't put in the permanent implants before radiation.

I pulled my pink bolero jacket tight around my chest and added up the months in my head. Chemo would take me up to mid-January, and radiation couldn't start until a month after that and would run six weeks. That took me to April. Four to six months after that meant late summer, almost a year out before I could get the permanent implants. Late summer meant the beginning of the new academic year, which meant I'd have to wait until December when I could take time off from work for the final surgery. That added a full year to the sprint-to-cancer-free schedule I'd been planning on.

I started to cry.

Jeff put his arm around me, and Ashley handed me a tissue. Dr. Smith patted my shoulder and said, we have to treat your cancer first. That's the most important goal here, to make sure you are cancer free. I know this is not what you wanted to hear, but none of this will be worth it if you're not cancer free.

I know, I know, I said. It's just not what I was expecting. It might take me a while to adjust.

Dr. Smith turned to the counter and scratched some notes in my chart while Ashley looked at me with sympathy, equipment tray clutched to her white exam coat. The air conditioning came on and blew my pink jacket open. I clutched it around me again, fumbling to hold it shut while swiping at my eyes.

Dr. Smith and Ashley left the room, Ashley handing me the tissues box on her way. Take it with you, she said. It's fine.

I took a fresh tissue and wiped my face. But I couldn't stop crying. I tried to pull myself together as I dropped the pink bolero jacket on the floor and pulled on my clothes, but I could barely see through my tears.

Ashley gave me a hug as I stumbled out of the office, and Jeff led me down the hall and out of the building into the fall sunshine. He helped me into the car, set the box of tissues on my lap, and shut the door with a thud. After he backed the car out of the parking space, he turned off the music, which was playing away with no regard for my distress, and pulled into traffic.

As Jeff drove us across town to the oncology clinic, I ranted through my tears. I'd made my way down this road, from a wee bit of cancer to a bilateral mastectomy to six freaking tumors, all the while thinking I could have most of it behind me by January. That's what Dr. Smith had told me in July. But that clearly was not going to be the case. Why was this happening? Why hadn't he warned me about this before the surgery? Why didn't the January mammogram, the multiple July mammograms, the MRI—any of them—show the extent of the cancer? Maybe I would have waited for the reconstruction and avoided this complication, this unknown path. I didn't want to adjust to one more unexpected twist. I just wanted it to be over as soon as possible.

I was still crying when we got to the oncology clinic.

I was starting to understand that cancer had taken over my life, and it would continue to dictate my life for the next year at least, and there was nothing I could do about it. It was time for another course correction, and it was devastating that it had to happen on my first day of chemo when I was already vulnerable and afraid. But there was no direction to go but forward.

•   •   •   •   •

At the oncology clinic, I was still crying when I took my seat amongst the balloons and the cookies, clutching the swag bag along with my box of tissues. I sat in the waiting room fuming, thinking furiously about popping some balloons. Jeff offered to fetch me things—cookies, tea, water, reading material—but I was too upset to respond.

Soon, Bonnie appeared and led us back to an exam room. Without comment, she took in my tears and the tissue box clutched in my hand and proceeded to measure my blood pressure and ask me about my pain level.

Preliminaries accomplished, Bonnie leaned back in her chair and said, it's not fair, is it?

No, I said through my tears. But it's not about that. Everyone says it's not fair. But for me, it's not about fairness. I know life isn't fair. I don't expect it to be fair. It's about feeling so helpless. What else could I have done? How else could I have lived my life to avoid this, to make it never happen? What did I do wrong?

Bonnie listened and let me sob, and Jeff listened and let me sob, and they both patted my arm and rubbed my back. But they had no answers because there are no answers. I was embarrassed to be crying on my first day of chemo because I didn't want anyone to think it was about chemo. Although I was terrified of chemo, I felt prepared for chemo and ready to be brave. But in that moment, I thought I would never again feel invincible, healthy, and confident that I was doing everything I could to live one hundred years and die peacefully in my bed.

At the time, I thought that was a loss I would never learn to live with. But now, at the other end of this ordeal, I've found some acceptance. We're all subject to forces beyond our control. Distracted or drunken drivers. Chemicals in our environment. Floods and earthquakes and rocks falling from the sun. You do the best you can to keep yourself and your family safe. And then you cope the best you can when the unexpected happens. I know now that even when the unexpected happened, I could still live in the light.

•   •   •   •   •

In the next hour, Dr. Chen reviewed my lab work, examined my extremities, and frowned at the state of my incisions. Then Bonnie handed me over to the nurses in the chemo room, who got me settled into the blue vinyl chair with the warm blankets, and Jeff went out to fetch lunch and cupcakes. My tears dried, as I was coming to know they would with each crisis, and I sat in the blue chair paging through Glamour Magazine, concentrating on fall style dos and don'ts. Jeff returned, and we ate our lunch and our cupcakes in peace, and waited for the poison to do its work.

Chemo infusions take time. Most of an afternoon, in fact. I had forgotten to take my anti-nausea steroid the night before, and they needed to run that first, so it would take even longer. During chemo, some people nap, some people watch TV or read, some people sit and chat with their support team. I did a little of each. You are perfectly functional while it's going on, which is partly why you think during that first infusion: this will be fine. A piece of cake, even if not one you want for your birthday.

Late in the afternoon, when all the poison was in, we drove home. On the drive, I started to feel a little dizzy, a little off, but not too bad. When we got home, I lay on the couch while Jeff and Elena accepted the food delivered for our dinner and set the table. This might not be so bad, I thought, as Elena told us about her day and I stroked the cat who had taken up residence on my belly. Dinner smelled pretty good.

I joined Jeff and Elena at the table to eat dinner. But halfway through, I realized I couldn't sit upright another minute. I was desperate to lie down, to escape the light and hide somewhere. I stumbled upstairs, pulling off my comfy shirt and my chemo pants, and fell into bed, oblivious to anything else around me. Jeff followed me upstairs and roused me enough that I could down some anti-nausea drugs with a glass of water. Then he turned out the lights and left me to sleep it off.

That's the thing about chemo. You think, oh this is going to be fine. I can take this. But a heavy, inescapable feeling, the fundamental opposite of physical well-being, creeps in on you, like a Victorian villain in a dark cloak following you down a foggy London block. As the villain darts from cranny to nook behind you, even as you glance over your shoulder and see nothing, your sense of dread rises, then rises some more, then even more, until suddenly the villain throws the cloak over you and bundles you into a carriage and spirits you off into the darkness. And once you are enshrouded in the dark cloak, you are so paralyzed that you can't even call out to your hero for rescue.

This is what surprised me about chemo: the dread. The dread happened even before I knew what to dread, before the nausea and leaden icky-ness took over. I felt as if chemo affected not only my physical body, but my very existential core. All I could do was enter the darkness and hunker down, waiting for whatever fate would befall me. It was an extremely physical feeling, as if every cell in my body wanted to shut down. But it was also deeply emotional, despairing. Not because I thought I was going to die. Rather, because I knew that the point was exactly the opposite: to keep me alive. Death was not the relief I could expect; there was no relief.

Some people try to convince you that chemo really isn't that bad these days because there are so many great anti-nausea drugs. So, they say, you don't have to suffer. That may be true for some, but it was not true for me. I suffered with chemo. I try not to see this as a moral failing. Maybe it would have been a lot worse without all the anti-nausea drugs, but it was bad enough with them.

During that first night, struggling to find relief from the nausea and the icky-ness, and inexperienced with the drugs, I took too many doses of something. Or maybe my soul just needed to detach from my poisoned body for a while. In any case, I can't remember anything about the next day, at least not as a normal perception. I know my sister Ann called, and I told her about chemo. I know Jeff drove me to the hospital for an injection to support my immune system, which I needed exactly twenty-four hours after chemo. But I retain only vague recollections of these events. The long hospital corridor accordion-pleating around me. Reclining in a blue vinyl armchair while a nurse chatted with Jeff and shot a large hypodermic into my arm. Listening to their voices as if I were in an echo chamber. Watching myself lie on the couch with a phone near my ear, but not understanding the words that came out of my own mouth. I know Bonnie called to check on me, but I don't remember talking to her.

Thursday, two days after chemo, I was better. By Friday, I was still a little dizzy and weak, and my guts were packed with cement. But I had a writing project due the next week, so I pulled myself together and wrote it, although I can't now figure out how I found the words. When I read that piece of writing now, I can't believe it came out of my brain during that week. It is completely rational and organized and coherent, and I felt anything but.

But I made it through that first chemo. And although I suffered, it wasn't for long. I can totally do this, I thought.

Chapter Thirteen

The Friday after my first chemo appointment was the day of the Big Flood in Northfield, an event that would pull anyone off their deathbed to walk downtown and take a look. Besides, I was feeling okay and ready to go out. So out I went.

The bucolic Cannon River winds through Northfield on its way to join the Mississippi near Red Wing, Minnesota. Native prairie grasses line the banks, a lushly green counterpoint to the flowing water, and mama ducks herd their babies along the shore. In the center of town, the river features a small waterfall, now a dam, which supplied power to the Malt-o-Meal cereal mill earlier in the town's history. Usually, it's a calm, canoe-able river, where the more daring ducks show off their paddling skills by drifting precariously near the lip of the falls, without ever going over. A few years ago, for the Fourth of July, some town boosters got together and raised enough money to shoot a human cannonball across the Cannon. The event brought out thousands of people to line the riverbanks and the bridges, although it was over in a few seconds.

Over the two days following my first chemo, it rained fifteen inches upriver from Northfield. The river rose and rose, then rose some more, until you could race kayaks in the riverside soccer fields and patrons drinking at the Froggy Bottom Pub had soggy bottoms. Classes at the colleges and the high school were suspended so strong-bodied youth could stack sandbags, and the National Guard came out to keep the public off the bridges.

Friday morning, testing my post-chemo legs, I wobbled the eight blocks to the river. This turned out to be the perfect chemo recovery activity: walk down to the river several times a day, check out the scene, and walk back. It got me out of the house for a little exercise, required no mental or emotional energy, and was mildly entertaining, but not over-stimulating. People brought their dogs and clutched them in their arms as they gazed together over the river wall at the roaring whitewater. The dogs apparently provided ballast against nature on a rampage, which I found odd.

After admiring the power of Mother Nature, to destroy but also to amaze, I would go home and curl up on the sofa again, where Ruby would put her head on my lap. I would stroke her velvet ears and scratch between her eyes while she sighed and closed her big brown eyes with pleasure. So, when it comes to the consolation of dogs, who am I to judge?

$$\bullet \qquad \bullet \qquad \bullet \qquad \bullet \qquad \bullet$$

Your hair starts to fall out about two weeks after your first chemotherapy. So the next week, my friend Sarah took me to strip-mall land, near the shop where I had purchased my supportive undergarments, to the wig place. I had decided to go with the wig, at least at work. I did not want to stand up in front of a class while wearing a constant reminder (e.g., a scarf or hat) that I was not functioning at one hundred percent. Teaching law students involves a certain kind of theater. You have to convince them that you have all the answers, and if they follow your lead and learn the rules of the game, they can be successful in this difficult enterprise. That's not guaranteed to be true, but they don't know that yet. You really just have to get them to settle down, have faith, and work hard. I didn't want a scarf to ding my credibility.

My sister Ruth, my sister-in-law Jody, and my friend Jackie are all exceptional needlewomen, and they had gone to work immediately and created a wardrobe of knitted and crocheted hats for me that would suit any ensemble or occasion. Jackie even knitted me a green and tan do-rag, which I wore once or twice, but which will mostly come in handy as part of some child's theater costume in the future. I decided that scarves were a little too chemo club for me, but that at home, hats would do perfectly well. Besides, the Minnesota winter was nigh, and wearing a hat inside full-time from October to March wouldn't raise a single eyebrow.

One friend argued for trying on an entirely new personality by getting entirely new hair. How about something long and blond, she said, or maybe red and curly? But if the point was to feel like myself professionally and avoid distracting my students, that didn't seem like a good idea. In retrospect, I think her suggestion was more about where she was in life, not me.

At just the right time, a neighbor who had gone through chemo a few years back kindly called to offer me advice about where to get a wig. At the time she went through cancer treatment, I wasn't even sure she was *having* chemo, even though someone asked me to pray for her at church, that's how good her wig was. So I decided to follow her advice.

Sarah and I trekked to the suburbs and found the wig place, DK International, in an industrial strip mall area, among kitchen cabinetry showrooms and obscure businesses with meaningless names like Protech and BSI. Driving by, you would not know it was a wig place. It could have been a business that shipped picture frames or sold frozen rodents as snake food. But having cancer teaches you many things about the world, like the fact that there are discreet businesses tucked away in industrial strip malls where you can get a circumspect, private wig fitting with a career wig expert. Where they will cut and style the wig for you and steam it to fit the shape of your head. Where you come out looking just like you looked when you went in, and your insurance company reimburses you for your trouble, and no one ever needs to know.

I still don't understand the secrecy around these matters. Cancer is nothing to be ashamed of. Losing your hair is nothing to be ashamed of. These are just circumstances that happen to us. Talking about cancer, or any other life challenge, does not jinx our recovery or make us less worthy as human beings. There are good reasons, as I had mine, for not wanting to parade around hairless, and everyone has to make the decision that works for them. But why does this business require a name like "DK International" rather than "Joe's Cancer Wigs"?

Anyway, I tried on wigs, and Sarah gave me a thumbs up or a thumbs down. Mary (!) the wig expert stood tactfully in the background, offering a considered opinion, but only when consulted. I ended up ordering "the Suzanne," which would perfectly match my existing short, salt-and-pepper hair once the wig was trimmed and shaped.

But there is no camouflage, no cover, for the hair you will lose elsewhere on your body. I'm not particularly hirsute, especially in the age of declining hormones. But I didn't realize before chemo that fine hair actually covers your entire body. It all fell out, more or less.

There was definitely an upside to this. During chemo, I had the smoothest, most wonderful skin I have ever had. My arms, legs, and face were as smooth as the proverbial baby's behind, like a nectarine when I'd always been a peach. But there was also a downside. I lost my nose hair, so I breathed essentially unfiltered air all day, drawing in dust and dirt and cat hair and pollen, and my sinuses couldn't keep up. Throughout chemo, my sinuses filled and bled and drained, which kept my neti-pot working overtime. And by the end of chemo, I had about a dozen eyelashes remaining, total for both eyes. Every morning, I carefully, optimistically plumped them up with mascara, but I still looked like a bit like a blue-eyed white rat.

And of course, there is pubic hair, which most of us don't want to talk about. But really—it's hair, and it is not exempt from the force that is chemo. I know Brazilian waxing and fancy pubic hair styling is popular these days, but I really hated feeling infantilized by this involuntary loss. And I never realized the service this hair provides. At a minimum, it protects certain sensitive parts of your body from the ravages of clothing friction, a not inconsiderable concern, I learned. I hear some people opt for the pubic hair wig, known as a merkin. But let's just not go there.

I went back to pick up the wig the next week, exactly on the day when my hair started to fall out in masses, carpeting my pillow in the morning and filling the sink. Mary, the wig expert, shaved what was left of my hair and then went off to steam the wig and fluff it up a bit.

At first, I hated the wig. I think I didn't actually believe this hair-loss thing would happen, and I still couldn't believe I had cancer, even though I now had Barbie boobs as a permanent reminder. I thought the wig looked ridiculous, that as I walked through the coffee shop, people would snigger behind shielding hands and whisper to their friends about the absurdity of trying to pretend I had hair. But I took it home, and when I modeled it that evening —for Jeff, Carolyn, and Elena—each of them, in turn, looked surprised and said, it's great. It looks just like your hair.

They were right. It did. When I look back at pictures taken during that time, I know I am wearing a wig. But you wouldn't know. And maybe, in time, I'll forget. Maybe years from now, I will look at pictures taken during late 2010 and early 2011 and have to check the photo data for the date, rather than know immediately: oh, that's 2010—I'm wearing the wig. In 2010, it seemed unlikely I would ever forget. But from here, I can just about imagine it.

In the mornings that next week and the weeks that followed, I put on my wig and brushed mascara on my thinning lashes and pulled my structured jacket over my fake breasts, and looked completely normal, even though my world was not normal and would not be normal again for a long time. And because Jeff leans towards the sexy Patrick Stewart look, we saved a bundle on shampoo that year.

•   •   •   •   •

I recognize now just how much I wanted my life during cancer to continue as normal. I wanted to look normal. I wanted to go to work and come home on my normal schedule. Essentially, I wanted to live my life unchanged by cancer.

Although I did my best to achieve these goals, and although I do believe that sticking as close to normal as possible brought me comfort, I'm not sure they were reasonable goals. Sometimes, normal is a lot to expect, and the expectation may be entirely self-imposed. I could have gone to work completely bald, and my students and colleagues would have adapted. I could have stayed in bed, day after day, and my family would have accepted my need to do that. I could have cried and wailed daily, not my normal pattern, and people would have been there to pass me the tissues. My need to be normal, I now believe, was about trying to control what was happening, which was not within my control.

If you are in the middle of this process, remember to live gently. Give yourself a break. While your usual response to crisis may be to soldier on, that's not the only response that will see you through. Don't be normal, if normal means operating 24-7, as it is for so many of us these days, and that's exhausting to you. You may feel okay between chemo sessions, but you have cancer. You're doing a big, courageous, difficult thing dragging yourself to the clinic every few weeks to siphon in the poison. That's not normal. So you don't have to stick to normal business hours, and you don't have to buck up, and you don't have to live your regular life. This probably seems obvious to everyone around you, but internalizing this message is a real challenge for some of us. I'm telling you: it's okay to let go.

Chapter Fourteen

A few months after I started chemo, a neighbor down the block in our old neighborhood discovered she also had stage III breast cancer.

Two data points make a pattern. What to make of this one? Were the gods moving through our neighborhood, smiting a woman in every sixth house to prove some inexplicable cosmic point? Or was it the houses? The houses in this neighborhood, built in the previous decade, were not high quality, environmentally sensitive structures. They were built to install families into the American Dream as cheaply as possible while leaving a tidy profit for the builder and minimizing the chance of collapse before the construction equipment cleared the site. The builder was ever so slightly shady, and I could imagine his company making a few extra bucks dumping toxic waste in the hole before cementing over the basement, or using illegal, black market adhesives to seal down the vinyl floors, which themselves exuded evil, noxious vapors.

It was easy to feel worse about Joanne's cancer than about my own. Joanne was in her mid-thirties and had six children, ranging in age from two (twin boys) to eight. Even if she survived it, her cancer would leave a permanent scar on the lives of those six children, who already ran a little wild in the cul-de-sac. As young adults, my children would be devastated to lose me, but they'd had a pretty unremarkable, stable childhood and would be fine no matter what. Who would provide that stability for Joanne's children, even for the year cancer would devour in her family's life?

I wanted to redirect all the casseroles and cakes and prayers her way. It seemed only fair. And I felt terrible that I was in no position to help. I couldn't even offer babysitting or housecleaning. I couldn't take this burden away from her, just as no one could take it away from me. I wanted to fix her, turn back the cellular process that dragged her here, her family trailing behind.

Besides, I barely knew her. What could I really do to help?

I realized that my family and friends must be in a similar place—feeling inadequate and ineffectual. How can a card, a meal, a phone call really make a difference? And yet I knew they did. So I sent Joanne a card that said, essentially, gosh this sucks. If you'd like to complain to someone who gets it, give me a call.

Joanne did call, and we had a good conversation about how our chemo was going and how her children were coping. I was glad to connect. I'm sure I couldn't really understand her experience because I didn't have to worry about my mortality while keeping six small children fed, clothed, and out of the street. But for a few minutes, I got to be on the other side of the equation, reaching out instead of looking in. It helped me internalize in a deeper way that this experience was about more than just me.

•　　　•　　　•　　　•　　　•

My chemo was scheduled for every three weeks, six sessions total. This intermittent schedule allows your body to recover, mostly, before it's poisoned again. Which is what keeps you alive, in theory.

Two weeks after my first session, I felt pretty good. In fact, I felt a burst of energy. I had recovered well from surgery and completed physical therapy—so I could shut the window and reach the salt—and I had resumed a reasonable work schedule. My wig and cap swaps became routine.

A languorous Minnesota fall unfolded, crisp and frosty in the mornings, warm and golden in the afternoons, with enough rain to keep the grass pliable under the eddies of leaves collecting on the lawn. In the air, the pungent smell of decay mixed with a little bit of smoke, an olfactory echo from childhood. At a local art fair, I bought a handmade African basket to mount on the handlebars of my upright townie bike. When I rode down the street under the flame-colored maples, I was twelve years old again, riding to my girlfriend's house to plan our Halloween get-ups. I considered inserting tinseled tassels into my handlebar grips, and I lifted my face into the breeze as I rode. My bike helmet collected dust in the garage. I figured I'd already had my brush with death. Life was good.

On the day of chemo two, Jeff and I visited Dr. Smith in the morning, where I got pumped up a few more ccs, then drove across town to the oncology clinic. Patient appreciation week was over, so there were no cookies or balloons in the lobby. At the reception desk, I popped a piece of hard candy into my mouth, anticipating the weird green onion taste that overwhelmed me when the lab tech flooded my chest port with saline. I was starting to know the routine.

Bonnie called us back to an exam room and asked the usual questions. She reported that my white blood counts had recovered remarkably well and that I was good to go. We chatted about our families—she has a daughter the same age as Elena—until she really needed to tend to other patients, then she gave me a hug and left. Dr. Chen came in, listened to my heart and lungs, examined my nails for trouble, smiled and nodded, and was on his way.

I started to feel a little nauseous before I even got to the chemo room, but I ate my lunch and settled in as the drip began. I had taken all the possible anti-nausea drugs ahead of time this round, and they seemed to hold me pretty well.

The morning after my initial chemo session, I had gone for acupuncture, to counter the chemo effects. I barely remembered it, and I wasn't sure it helped, but I had made another appointment to follow this second session. So when the drip was done, we headed right to the acupuncture clinic, where I spent an hour with needles sticking out of my knees. We drove home in the dark, and I refused dinner and proceeded directly to bed. I was up in the night to take more anti-nausea drugs, but I slept pretty well and awoke feeling positive and reasonably functional.

Over the next few days, I stayed home and recovered. Elena was off school for fall break, so I had company. And while I know I had the same couple days of icky-ness and nausea as with the first round, it didn't seem that bad. Maybe the acupuncture helped. Maybe I was learning how to use the drugs to best effect. Maybe I was adapting and not feeling so anxious about the whole process. Jeff and I resumed our hiking on Sunday morning, a few days later, and I emerged from the weekend thinking I could totally do this.

Perhaps the earlier dread, as physical as it seemed, was about not knowing. Going into the first chemo, I didn't know if I could work and do chemo at the same time. I didn't know how many days I would be laid out in bed and how many days I would feel normal-ish. I didn't know if I would be able to walk the dog and cook dinner and grade papers and drive the hour to work and back and be a parent to my children. Now it seemed I could expect to be laid out for a few days, but not too many. My life was not completely suspended during this time if I kept a reasonable pace.

I could have cried with relief.

•   •   •   •   •

For several years after I completed my cancer treatment, when I opened a bathroom drawer or rooted around in the hall closet for the button box, I still encountered the detritus of cancer. Chemo makes your tubes shut down, and, really, the body is an intricate set of tubes, which keep the vital fluids moving from place to place, like the interstate highway system tangled up with the Mississippi River and the Burlington Northern Railroad. And when there's major road construction on I-80 and a drought on the river and a train wreck to boot, moving the goods is a challenge. Similarly, during chemo, your tubes may need a little extra lubrication or locomotion assistance, just to keep functioning.

Jars and vials and boxes of remedies cluttered my cupboards and drawers. There were drugs to treat urinary tract infections because my body couldn't fight infections. Anti-yeast tablets and various tubes of anti-itching cream, because fungus loves a depressed immune system, and about twelve different constipation remedies. During chemo, I took them all—at the same time, along with my whole grain, oatmeal-prune cookies and applesauce and my gallons of water. There was magic mouthwash—the actual technical name for it—used to treat the sores that develop in your mouth during chemo. There was a bundle of catheters tied up in an orange rubber band, for when that particular tube *really* didn't want to work, and half a dozen different nausea remedies, which I popped like candy for a while, plus three pairs of anti-nausea acupressure wristbands.

All this crowded alongside bottles of hydrocodone, oxycodone, and muscle relaxants. It's great that there's so much attention on treating pain, but really. Every time I had the most minor procedure, I was handed another prescription for fifty or so tablets. The drugs made me sicker than the pain ever did, so I would take a few, then stash them away. I considered financing an early retirement on the street value but eventually took them to the city's drug disposal box.

In the hall cabinet, there were Neti pots and boxes of Neti salts, because the sinuses are also basically a tube and are not exempt from inflammation. They move a lot of freight in the form of air. Plus, once your nose hair falls out, the tracks are kind of rusty. The Neti pots clattered around with the various-sized Aquaphor tubes and the giant bottle of aloe used to soothe irradiated flesh, which might otherwise peel off like the skin of a well-barbequed chicken. Aquaphor doubles as great lip gloss, so I'm set for life in that department.

In my dresser drawer, there was a tube of KY Jelly and a bottle of Glide Personal Lubricant. Because, believe it or not, you may still be thinking about having a sex life despite your treatment and its horrors, even though it takes some creative thinking and a partner who still believes you're the bees' knees. My gynecologist later recommended throwing out the KY and Glide and substituting coconut oil. Or better yet, a tub of Crisco, the latest gynecological lubricant of choice. I am now unable to make pie crust without thinking about this. Another unanticipated side effect of cancer.

For over a year after chemo, in my kitchen pantry, I had four kinds of ginger ale, several kinds of ginger candy, ginger tablets, ginger tea, and ginger cookies. A dear friend had contributed this collection, convinced that something had to help.

At this point, a couple years after cancer, I knew I should just toss everything in a bag and pitch it in my not-pink trash bin for Dick's Sanitation to haul away on Monday morning. But I didn't. Maybe I was afraid I would need it again soon. That throwing it out would tempt Fate, invite that unyielding bitch to turn around and shower me again with the magic pink sparkle dust that gave me cancer in the first place. Maybe continuing to let the tubes and bottles and boxes inhabit my storage space was a way to humble myself to Fate, hoping she'd be kind.

•   •   •   •   •

Chemo three about killed me.

When I look back at it, I think I did everything wrong. Hubris, I guess. Two data points make a pattern, right? Everything had gone so well in September and October, with the balmy weather and the golden afternoons and the return to regular life after the hoopla of diagnosis and surgery and recovery. Despite the trouble with tubes, I dared to think all could be normal, that I was the stronger party in this battle. David with my slingshot. A Greek in a wooden horse, poised to conquer the mighty city of Troy.

Chemo three was scheduled for the first Thursday in November. I was busy at work and could not have chemo on Tuesday and take the rest of the week off, as I had done for chemo one and two. I pushed the appointment to Thursday afternoon, so I would only have to miss one work day that week. Surely, I thought, I would be ready to go back to work on Monday now that I knew what I was up against.

Early in the week, I told Jeff it would be totally fine for him to skip going to chemo with me this time. And it would be totally fine for me to put in that full day of work before I went to chemo. And it would be totally fine to spend the next two days at home by myself, since he and Elena both had commitments elsewhere, and to skip the acupuncture since Jeff couldn't take me.

Maybe I went into that session more tired and stressed, struggling to meet self-imposed, unreasonable expectations. Maybe I should not have been alone, when I'd been good about accepting help up to now. Maybe the acupuncture actually helped. Maybe it was just time for me to confront my grief.

Whatever the reason, the day after chemo session three, I crashed. Alone in the silent house that morning, I made my way downstairs, but felt a leaden sickness settle in, more weighty than anything I'd experienced with the previous two sessions. I tried to get comfortable for the day. I closed the blinds to protect my aching head from the dim November sunlight, then hunkered down on the brown sofa and pulled a quilt to my chin.

Comfortable was not possible. Over the next several hours, my body burned and ached and refused to move, and I could find no relief. It felt as though all my cells were trying to escape some catastrophe, ready to jump ship if only they could. All I could do was enter the darkness and await my fate, like a wounded animal.

I lay on the sofa, unable to crawl upstairs to my bed, and watched streaks of light filter through the blinds and inch across the wall. Ruby lay on the floor next to me, her nose on her paws, somehow understanding that I could not get up to let her out into the bracing November air, which she would have preferred. I didn't have the energy to reach down and stroke her head, or to swat the cats away as they hovered on the back of the sofa, or to point the remote towards the TV. I turned my head to vomit into the aluminum bowl we keep especially for that purpose, but then couldn't get up to empty it. It sat on the coffee table, stinking up the room with its contents.

And I began to wonder. Why *had* I survived that near-death fall last spring? What was I hanging on for? My children were nearly grown. If I died, my spouse would move on. I was just another data point in a universe of a million human data points. None of us was that important. If I chose not to suffer like this again, my decision would make hardly a ripple out there in the larger world.

I shut my eyes and tried not to think.

Around five o'clock, Jeff came home. He saw me on the sofa, the overflowing bowl on the table next to me, and dropped his bags. I cracked open an eye and looked at him.

I can't do this, I said. I would rather die than feel like this again.

I started to cry.

He sat down next to me on the sofa and put a hand on my leg.

Tell me, he said.

As I cried, I told him how terrible I felt, and how I had tried to be brave through everything, but couldn't do it anymore, and how I didn't care what happened to me. Live or die, I just wanted it to stop.

He patted my leg while I cried, and I somehow mustered the energy to wail and rage, until I had nothing left. Then he emptied the putrid bowl, fetched the tissues and a glass of water, and helped me sit up so I could sip it.

You don't have to do anything you don't want to do, he said, as I gulped down tears and sipped my water. But give it one more session. For me. For the kids. If you want to stop after that, okay. But don't decide right now. Now is not the time.

Then he helped me upstairs and put me to bed.

So I didn't decide. I would give it some time. But I wasn't promising anything.

•   •   •   •   •

Over the next week, I returned to something like normal. But I dreaded the next chemo date. I shouldn't fear the suffering, I thought. I should want to live, no matter what. But at night, I lay awake, wondering if I had the courage to keep going.

I decided I could not make it through six sessions of chemo. But I promised Jeff I would do four—one more and I was done. Damn the turbulent waters, I thought. Let's see where I land.

I decided to pull out all the stops, just so I could survive that one session. And there remained only one stop to be pulled: illegal drugs.

I was never much of an experimenter in my youth. I drank too much a couple times in college, but mostly I prefer my reality boring and unaltered, neurotic though it may be. But I figured there must be a reason why in some states, you can get the Big J to treat the Big C. And if I had to choose between feeling like I would rather die than do chemo again and breaking a few laws, I would choose breaking the law.

I thought a long time about this decision. Lawyer jokes aside (Q: What is a criminal lawyer? A: Redundant.), I take the good moral character requirement imposed on licensed attorneys seriously. After all, for a while, I wrote a professionalism column for a law student publication. As a law professor, I considered myself a role model for my students. I try not to speed. I don't drive when I've had a glass of wine. But now, weighing the considerations, alleviating suffering took precedence.

How, then, does one go about obtaining such a substance? And what does one do with it once it is in hand? I needed to do some research.

Of course, I could have asked Sam. He was a college student, and I'd be fooling myself if I thought he didn't at least know who to ask on campus. But I didn't want to put him in the position of performing an illegal act for his mother. That seemed like a boundary transgression, like requiring a ten-year-old to arrange and pay for his own birthday party. Bad Mother.

So instead, I brought it up with some friends. And they came through, as they always did. I have a friend, let's call her Mary since everyone else is named Mary, who is an upstanding member of the community and an exceptionally moral person. She goes to church and participates in church-lady activities, like delivering meals to old people and baking bread for communion. She works with children and won't even jaywalk in town lest someone see her and get the wrong idea. She walks to work, even in the cold, to minimize her environmental footprint. And she offered to get me some pot.

I was scheduled for chemo number four the day before Thanksgiving. I didn't know how or when — or really whether — this transaction would happen. But I didn't want to bother my friend for details, in case she had changed her mind.

On Sunday night before Thanksgiving, around 9 p.m., the doorbell rang. I pulled myself off the brown sofa and headed to the door, wondering who would come by at what was, for us, such a late hour. Sam wouldn't be home from school until Tuesday, so it couldn't be one of his friends. And Elena was out studying for a pre-break physics test.

I flipped on the porch light and peered through the transom window into the flood of greenish light. I vaguely recognized the young woman standing on the steps with her hands shoved deep in her pockets, but I wasn't sure. An unfamiliar young man stood behind her. We live in Northfield, so criminal ambush seemed an unlikely possibility. I opened the door.

Hi, said the young woman. I'm Anna. Mary's daughter?

Oh my gosh, I said, opening the door wide. I barely recognized you. I haven't seen you for probably four years, since you graduated from high school. How are you? Come in.

I'm fine, she said, stepping inside and bringing the cold November air with her. The young man stepped in behind her. I caught a glimpse of the Big Dipper glittering above the neighbor's house as I shut the door.

This is my boyfriend, Josh, she said, motioning with her head. She pulled a plastic bag out of her pocket and held it out to me.

My mom said you needed this.

I took the bag and examined it in the dim light filtering through the window from the porch. It looked exactly like the supply of oregano I had put up in my pantry the previous summer.

My god, I thought. I'm engaging in my first ever illegal drug transaction. If Jeff were here, I would have him take a picture. I refrained from calling him to the door.

I live down the hall from my college's main drug dealer, Anna said. We're home for the week since it's Thanksgiving. So you have good timing.

She smiled.

Wow, I said, turning the bag over in my hand. Thank you. I don't know if it will help, but I SO appreciate you being willing to do this for me. I'm really excited to try it.

I hugged her.

Lame, I thought. I am so lame. What is the protocol for middle-class, middle-aged lady drug deals?

No problem, she said. It's pretty easy to get this stuff on campus. Mom would have brought it over, but we wanted to get out of the house.

We determined that I owed her $40. Anna and Josh petted the dog and exclaimed about how fluffy she was while I went to get the cash. Maybe, I thought as I fetched the money, my attorney ethical principles will be intact if Jeff pays for it. I took the money out of his wallet.

I had no idea how to turn the contents of the bag into something I could consume. But I decided it would be asking too much to invite Anna and Josh to demonstrate. So I handed over the $40, thanked them profusely once again, and wished them a happy Thanksgiving as I waved them out the door.

In the previous week, I had learned how easy it is to get the accessories you need to smoke pot, although the accessories did not come with instructions. Somehow, I didn't think to Google for rolling instructions. But to get the accessories, you Google what you need, type in your credit card number, and wait for your package to arrive in the mail. I ended up with enough rolling paper to supply Northfield High School for a couple of months, because it's a bargain when you buy in bulk on the Internet, and my mother taught me to never pass up a bargain.

The next day, I sent out a cry for help, and the night before my chemo appointment, a friend came over to show me how to roll a joint. I'd lived in the house for six months, and for the first time, I shut the blinds in the living room, lest the police drive by and somehow discern that our huddle around the kitchen island was for illegal purposes, not to sample the pecan pie. I made sure Elena was tucked up in her room for a while, and then my friend lined up five white rectangles of paper and sprinkled a generous line of weed down the center of each while the cats sniffed expectantly at the plastic bag. My friend rolled several expert joints—big fat babies that she assured me should do the job. I fumbled with mine, spilling stray seeds and sticks on the floor. The dog came over to investigate the spillage, but ultimately turned up her nose and went to lie down under the table.

Later, I squirreled away my little stash—in my underwear drawer, where else?—and waited for the moment when I would call on Puff to help me face the turbulent sea.

•　　　•　　　•　　　•　　　•

At the oncology clinic reception desk that Wednesday morning, I popped a hard candy into my mouth to offset the coming green onion taste, then waited to be put through my paces. I submitted to the port flushing and the blood draw, then the weighing and measuring, then took a seat in the exam room, Jeff at my side, as usual. My heart pounded the whole time.

In the exam room, Bonnie covered the preliminaries, including my difficulties after the previous session, the state of all my tubes, and my remarkably resilient white blood cells. Then she sat back and asked me how I was, really.

That last chemo just about killed me, I said. I'm not sure I can get through six. I promised Jeff I would come today and do this one more. But can we at least talk about what happens if I want this to be my last chemo? How do the statistics change if I stop at four?

Bonnie looked at Jeff, then back at me.

That worries me, she said. But yes. We can talk about that. I'll get Dr. Chen.

She patted my shoulder on her way out of the room.

I relaxed. This was the right response. She did not try to talk me out of it. She did not pooh-pooh my misery. In those few words, she recognized that I was suffering and that I needed her to take my suffering seriously. I probably changed my mind about skipping chemo five and six right then, wanting to live because Bonnie was on my side.

But the next few minutes were when I wished I'd been more proactive about finding a doctor I connected with. In a crisis of confidence, the moment when you must decide whether the cost is worth the outcome, you need information. And you need compassion. And you need someone to witness your suffering and help you through the door to the next treatment because you are not sure you can do it alone.

But when Dr. Chen entered the room, he listened briefly to my question, then responded like this: You have really bad cancer. You need six chemos.

I'm sure there is research to shore up the conclusion that I needed six chemos. But that's not what I was asking. Besides some compassion about my suffering, I wanted data to help me make a decision. I wanted to know how much two more sessions of chemo improved my chances. Would four chemo mean I *might* still die, but probably not? Would six chemo mean I definitely would not? Would four mean: you'll see next

Christmas, but don't count on the following? Would six mean: meet the grandchildren? What about five? Would five mean I'd get to fifty, but shouldn't count on Elena's college graduation, still five years away?

I don't know if Dr. Chen could have answered these questions for me. I'm not sure if there is research to show how much difference two more sessions make, or one more, or three more. But he didn't try to answer, and I regret not pushing him. Not shouting and crying and demanding information that would help me decide to live.

Since then, I've read conflicting information about whether chemo actually increases your chances of survival by a significant percentage. So I wonder what would have happened had I refused more sessions. Most of us, I think, subject ourselves to this horror without enough information because we are, in fact, so desperate to live. Chemo is awful, so how can it not make you better? Why would anyone ask you to undergo this torture if it didn't save your life? And I don't want to think too much about it now, because I regret not choosing my doctor more carefully and regret not standing up for myself on that day. I didn't do my best, and I'm embarrassed about that.

So I soldiered into the chemo room and sank into the blue chair, averting my eyes as the nurse hung the grapefruit dish soap bag on the IV line so I would not start gagging any sooner than necessary. Jeff held my hand as the drip began. I picked at my lunch, then dozed in the blue chair, listening to the nurses discuss their Thanksgiving plans, believing this might be the final Thanksgiving for me.

This is it, I thought. I am done. I am not doing this again.

Deciding that this was my last chemo got me through that day. When we got back to town, I had my acupuncture session, then went home, where I tossed down a handful of anti-nausea drugs, including a little Ativan, because what the hell, and went to bed. I slept well, knowing I was done with chemo, whatever Dr. Chen thought.

•   •   •   •   •

I dreaded the following day, when I expected the unendurable malaise to ambush me again. Jeff's family had offered to cook the holiday meal and bring it to our house in Northfield. So I could stay upstairs away from the hubbub if I needed to, but I would not be alone for the day. I figured I couldn't smoke the pot while the family was there. So in the morning, I remained curled up in bed, sleeping on and off, and waiting for the full impact of chemo to hit me. The sounds of family arriving and the clinking and clanking of dinner preparations filtered up the stairs, infecting my dreams, making me restless.

Midday, I awoke and realized that I didn't yet feel as sick as I expected. But I lay there feeling isolated and sorry for myself anyway, unwilling to join the crowd. I thought about how much I wanted the day to be normal, with all the normal family irritations and pleasures. I wanted to score the big win on the Family Bingo card when Uncle Ted told the story about the dead squirrel again, or Cousin Jim spilled the wine, as usual. I wanted to gossip with my sister-in-law in the kitchen while we peeled potatoes. I wanted to play dumb word games and groan about too much food after dinner. I did not want to mix in this complication—me being stupidly ill—which would make people pity me and feel like they should fetch me things and take care of me. Besides, I knew I could not get through the pre-dinner "This year I'm thankful for . . ." without crying.

So I dozed off again. But from my bedroom, I began to smell turkey roasting and gravy simmering. Soon, a suggestion of warming pies and caramelizing vegetables mingled with the turkey. As I came around, I realized the aroma of food did not make me feel ill, as I expected. I was actually hungry. I lay there a few minutes watching the crows squabble on the icy branches outside my window. Then I got up, washed my face, pulled my favorite red hat onto my bald head, and went downstairs.

They had set me a place at the table, just in case. I inserted myself between Elena and Jeff and accepted a small serving of turkey, mashed potatoes, and gravy. It tasted pretty good, so I had a little more. Then I had a little more. Then I had some pie, and a little more pie, because we always have three kinds—pecan, apple, and French silk—and who can choose, really? The girls sang show tunes at the piano while Uncle Rick and the boys cleaned up the mess. We all slipped the dog turkey scraps when we thought no one else was looking. Everyone told a lot of road-worn stories, but some new ones too.

And I was very thankful, but I didn't cry. Surrounded by my family, my back warmed by the fire in the hearth, I knew that even if more suffering awaited me, I wanted to be here for every possible minute.

Chapter Fifteen

After that, my recovery from chemo four went surprisingly well. I lazed around the rest of Thanksgiving weekend, nibbling away at the turkey and potatoes, cutting another tiny sliver off the French silk pie, happy to miss the shopping crowds. The academic term had finished up before the holiday, so I had papers to grade, but nothing more taxing on my agenda. Which may explain why I abandoned the idea of skipping chemo five and six. If five and six were as easy as four, I decided, I could commit to the "meet my grandchildren" plan.

The fact is, I never smoked the pot. A year later, in the month before Sam had his colon out, when he was trying every last-ditch Crohn's disease remedy before surrendering to the heartbreaking choice to remove his colon at age twenty-one, I gave it to him.

Here, I said. Try this. Maybe it will help.

Maybe that was a boundary violation even greater than asking him to find me a dealer. But at the time, it felt like what any mother would do. I think he went out one frigid December night and smoked it with a college friend. I'm sure it did wonders for both their colons.

•   •   •   •   •

In December, my sister Jane came to keep me company during the fifth chemo process. Outside of the chemo three period, with its hubris-induced misery, Jeff and I had been keeping the household running, what with the meals delivered three times a week, friends looking in on us regularly, and Elena hanging out at home a lot, working on her calculus and her physics, to a background of *Veronica Mars*. But another pair of hands, and just the company, was welcome during those few days surrounding chemo. So I was grateful when Jane offered to come.

At this point, chemo felt routine. It's not that the effects got easier, although I never again descended into quite the abyss that chemo three induced. But we were on the downhill side of the mountain, so anything bad that happened could only happen once more, which seemed easy enough to deal with. And I think you really do learn to manage your drugs and your bowels and your expectations so you can get through it.

Just two more times. Just one more time.

Chemo five was memorable because it began the long series of Dr. Smith's Cut and Stitch Parties, which went on for about the next year. I had finished getting "fills" at Dr. Smith's office sometime in October, so I now proudly sported temporary C cup boobs that filled out my pre-surgery wardrobe quite nicely. But in December, at the exam before chemo five, Dr. Chen prodded the surgical incision on my right side with a gloved finger. Two pea-sized splits in the seam remained, exposing the fake-derma-corpse tissue underneath.

He tutted reflectively, poked several other places on my melon-firm breast, and said, "Too much fill. Who's your surgeon?" He left the room to confer with Bonnie, who was charged with calling Dr. Smith's office to review the situation.

The chemo drip began, and it was lovely sitting and catching up with Jane rather than chatting inanely with the nurses for another three hours, as pleasant as they always were. Jeff went to get our usual lunch of gourmet salads from a nearby cafe, and we passed the afternoon in the blue vinyl chairs, with the usual agenda of chatting, naps, and reading. But mid-afternoon, Bonnie came back to the chemo room to deliver the news that we needed to trek back across town to Dr. Smith's office when we were done with the chemo, so he could take a look at the incision. He had agreed to stay at the office as long as it took. Because that's the kind of guy he is. And that's why he gets rated as one of the best plastic surgeons for women every year in the local magazine poll. It's really not just about his looks.

So at five o'clock, we piled into the car and set off across town in rush hour traffic. And indeed, Dr. Smith and Ashley were both at the office waiting for us when we got there forty-five minutes later. They took me back to a procedure room, where I donned the pink paper gown and settled onto the exam table. Jeff came with me, just in case. In case of what, I'm not sure. But I was getting better at saying yes, so I didn't protest.

Dr. Smith first stuck a needle through the expander valve on the right side and extracted several ccs of saline, so for the next few months I would list to the left a bit and need to stuff tissues into my right bra cup to even things up if I wore a t-shirt. Next, he swabbed the area with betadine, shot in a little Novocain, even though I could feel nothing, and carefully cut around the unhealed incision. I could feel the blood trickling down my chest and smell the sharp, antiseptic scent of the betadine. Ashley stood sentry, ready to mop up the stray fluids as best she could. I concentrated once again on the candlelit yoga studio, where I was missing my regular Tuesday night class. Jeff looked on from his chair in the corner while Dr. Smith stitched me up again, plastered me with steri-strips and gauze, snapped off his gloves, and patted my foot. It was about 6:30.

Let's see you in a week, he said, and make sure this is healing okay. This is the kind of thing that keeps me up at night.

I always believed his remarks like that. It made me feel like he totally deserves his $5000 an hour. *I didn't have to lie awake worrying. He* would do it on my behalf. Maybe it was just his patter, but isn't that what you want to believe about your doctor?

When I went back the next week so he could take a look, it was in fact healing well, seams knitting tightly, keeping my insides where they should be. So I sailed towards my final chemo, confident that all would soon be well.

Chapter Sixteen

The hurdle between chemo five and chemo six was Christmas. When you have cancer, you think a lot about whether this will be your last _____ (fill in the blank). We planned to join my family at my sister Jane's house in Texas for five days, traveling on Christmas Eve. So besides worrying about whether this would be my last Christmas, I worried about whether it would be the last time I saw some of my family, all of whom I adore. The kids had blossomed into adulthood and suddenly had lives of their own. In the next few years, they would acquire jobs and in-laws and children, or maybe not have the means for holiday travel every year. I lay awake at night imagining that the next family gathering would be my funeral, and I'd miss all the fun, not to mention the cake.

On the morning of December 23, as we were wrapping up the cookie baking and starting to consider packing for the trip, Sam pulled up his shirt and asked, what do you think about this rash?

I looked at his side, where a patch of angry, weeping sores was starting to creep from his stomach around towards his spine.

This Christmas trip is doomed, I thought.

I think that rash looks nasty, I said. Does it hurt? Does it itch?

It hurts some, he said. And I'm not feeling that great.

I think you need to get it checked out, I said. How about Dad takes you to the clinic while I finish up these cookies?

So Jeff, ever ready to sit in another clinic chair for however long it took, drove Sam to urgent care, while Elena and I stayed home and pressed colored sprinkles into frosting.

The rash was shingles. Standard treatment for Crohn's Disease is immunosuppression, and immunosuppression makes the body susceptible to illnesses young people would otherwise never contract. Despite the anti-shingles medicine prescribed that morning at the clinic, the rash got progressively worse, and soon Sam couldn't do much more than lie on the sofa (his sofa was the green one with the kitty blanket;

my sofa was the brown one with the red afghan) and watch *Burn Notice*, his current stupid TV of choice. Fortunately, he wasn't in a lot of pain, unlike many shingles sufferers, but he felt terrible and clearly shouldn't travel. So Jeff once again got on the phone with the airline and negotiated a ticket wrangle. This time, the airline was willing to issue credit in the amount of purchase for future use (Merry Christmas?). But we didn't know how the symptoms would progress for Sam, so we couldn't make a catch-up plan for later in the week.

The next day, Christmas Eve, Elena and I caught the afternoon flight to San Antonio without Jeff and Sam, leaving me wondering if I would spend my last Christmas without even my nuclear family around me. Jeff promised they would follow in a few days if Sam felt up to it, but I felt unsettled and torn leaving them behind. Once again, two major illnesses in one family put us in a particularly painful position. But we had to decide, so we split up.

In later years, I would see how these difficult decisions affected our family. Despite our efforts to cushion Elena from the vagaries of two major illnesses, she would end up feeling untended. Our nuclear family became unpracticed in spending time together, a skill we might have to develop later. Jeff and I would carry the guilt of having to choose where to put our resources, which were abundant, but not unlimited. It was hard. Sometimes we had only bad choices, it seemed. We did the best we could, all the while wishing we could do better.

•   •   •   •   •

As Elena and I completed the car rental transaction in San Antonio, we joked nervously about the super-sketchy off-site rental facility, something I never worried about when we traveled as a family. But during this period, I always figured that no one would mess with a woman with cancer. If worse came to worse, I could always pull off my hat, yank up my shirt, and say, look—do you really want to prey on a dying woman? As long as we didn't encounter a psychopath, I figured we were fine.

We got into the rental car, then pulled onto the highway for the short drive to Jane's house. It began to rain, Texas style. It rained so hard that by the time we got off the highway ten minutes later and started the trek across city streets, the street was running like a river. I thought I'd had my baptism into healing with the Northfield flood earlier in the fall, but maybe I needed another dose, just to make sure. Maybe it was like needing six chemo—several symbolic cleansings were required, because my cancer was, well, bad. Once again, I resorted to a kind of magical thinking. If I endured enough biblical flooding, I would be cured. If I navigated just one more obstacle, I would be safe.

We traversed the flooded streets to Jane's house, where we fell into the warm embrace of my family. They took good care of me, and I didn't even mind letting them. If it turned out this was my last Christmas, I couldn't ask for more. Sam improved quickly, so he and Jeff were able to travel on the 26th, which completed the circle.

Two events stuck with me from that week. First, during the pre-dinner family circle on Christmas night, where we check in and sing a song of some sort, more or less our substitute for a prayer, my niece Abby offered that she had dedicated her yoga practice to me that day, to send me healing energy. I adore Abby, and I was extremely touched, so I lost it, of course, and started sobbing, something I had sworn I wouldn't do. And then my mother lost it, and Elena lost it, and some of my sisters and nieces, and then we were all in a huddle sobbing, acknowledging my state in a way we hadn't in the twenty-four hours since I arrived.

I really appreciated this thoughtfulness from Abby. It's hard to gauge at a family gathering like this how much to talk about your cancer and the peculiar experiences you are having. I was spending most of my time thinking about cancer or dealing with cancer or doing things to promote my healing from cancer, and I didn't have a lot else to talk about. Unless you wanted to talk about Crohn's Disease. Cancer was my project, my current life's work, my career. But you really don't want to spend five days talking only about cancer. So how much to bring it up? Should you bring it up at all? Abby named it as real.

But someone else told me later they thought this announcement was awkward and unnecessary and took the family to a place we didn't need to go. I didn't experience it that way, but maybe so. Maybe doing anything that calls attention to the fact of cancer, which also causes the cancer subject to cry, or anyone else to cry, should be avoided. This just shows how differently people can feel about cancer and how hard it is to Do the Right Thing.

Second, later in the week, Jane arranged for a massage therapist to come to her teaching studio (she's an artist) and provide massages to whoever wanted them. I love massage and was first in line. So at two o'clock that afternoon, I stripped, climbed onto the heated table, and pulled up the cotton blanket. The therapist was an older woman with New Age leanings. She offered some regular massage and some healing touch, which did not always involve actual touch.

As the therapist hovered over me, she began to talk about my "wings"—how she could feel them sprouting in my energy field, mid-back. I should let my wings flourish, she advised, so they could grow strong and carry me to the next phase of my destiny. I shouldn't worry, she said, I was on the course meant for me.

Despite my struggle to believe in anything I can't see tangible evidence of, I don't mind talk like this normally, because what do I know? Not much. Normally, I think it doesn't hurt anything, whether I believe it or not. But this "sprouting wings" soliloquy led me down only one path: Angels. Can wings mean anything other than angels, and can angels mean anything other than death?

Of course, the value of an intuitive perception like this lies in what the receiver makes of it. In fact, the following Christmas, when I was indeed not dead, one of the nieces brought an animal totem encyclopedia along to the family gathering, and we all spent hours contemplating our animal totem options. For various reasons, including the fact that bald eagles seemed to follow me around the week my father died in 2007, I decided mine was a bald eagle. Bald eagles are intuitive, watchful, and powerful, but have relatively weak voices. So they appeal to my aspiration to be a good listener and a quiet leader, in touch with my inner power, but at the same time, they give a nod to my occasional timidity about speaking up.

Deciding to adopt the bald eagle as my totem animal, and placing tiny plastic bald eagles in strategic locations (my desk, my dresser) as a reminder to feel my power and use my voice, actually helped me make some big life and career decisions over the following year. So maybe the massage therapist had been completely right—I was sprouting wings. I was the one who leapt to the conclusion that they were angel wings, and, consequently, that I was going to die. Maybe they were bald eagle wings all along, and if I had decided that in December 2010, I would have saved myself some trouble.

When you are in the cancerland jungle, everything seems to relate back to cancer. But it doesn't have to. Even when you're suffering through surgeries and chemotherapy and radiation, you still have a life and a future, even if you don't know how long that future stretches ahead. Sometimes wings are eagle wings, there to carry you forward into the next phase of actually living your life. So fuck the angels, even if they come to you at Christmas.

•   •   •   •   •

Chemo six, the week after the holidays, was a piece of cake, more or less. I suffered in the usual ways, but it was the end, so I could tolerate anything. Afterward, I was sprung, released, set free, liberated. If I owned a gun, I would have shot it recklessly into the air until I exhausted my ammunition. Think fireworks and brass bands and little girls in frilly white dresses waving flags.

The semester didn't start for two more weeks, and Jeff had planned a mid-January celebratory trip to Florida, where we would walk on the beach, eat delicious Cuban food, and soak up some natural radiation for a few days. Treatment radiation, which would start at the end of the month, would take time from my daily routine. But, I was told, it would probably not challenge me physically the way chemo had. I could see the home stretch from here.

So I sat in the abundant sun on Lido Key Beach, a safe distance from the current pulling at the shore, and felt my bleeding sinuses begin to heal in the sea air. I burrowed my bare feet into the warm, sugary sand, and I let the rhythm of the waves rock me into a new life.

Chapter Seventeen

After chemo, you start to wonder if you can now reenter the land of the living. Sure, radiation is up next, but it won't be nearly the ordeal of chemo. So the worst is over. Is this the time to move out of emotional purgatory and decide you no longer have cancer? Or should you wait? When exactly *do* you no longer have cancer? When the nurses look you in the eye again? When you have not fallen down for a year?

Although I struggled with these questions in that liminal period between chemo and radiation, I could pretty much resume my regular life. My hair would start to grow back about twelve weeks after my last chemo, or so I was told. We declined further Sunday, Tuesday, and Thursday meal deliveries, and I resumed cooking. But at some point, I had to decide in my head that I no longer had cancer. That the olly-olly-oxen-free call sent out to those errant cells had actually worked. That they had heeded the call, headed back to base, and been tagged out. Except maybe a few sneaky, delinquent ones still lurked behind the shed, like that weird kid from the neighborhood who nobody wanted to play with, but who joined the game anyway and wouldn't go home. Maybe that one would wait in the shadows, concealed beneath the thick, prickly arms of the spirea bush until dark, and then ambush me again when I least expected it.

I walked Ruby in the dark January mornings, regaining my strength, careful of the ice glazing the sidewalks, and stood by to learn from her exuberance as she dove headfirst into snowdrifts and rolled around ecstatically on her back. And I began a morning walk mantra that I try to repeat every morning even now: Just one more day. Just one more day. By that I mean: no matter when I die, whether it's tomorrow or in ten years or in forty years, no matter how much I'm suffering or how much I fear what comes next, I am grateful for one more day, and I will do my best to honor that day.

• • • • •

Thirty-three sessions. Every weekday. 3:20 p.m. Those are my radiation statistics. Six weeks and three days, then I could graduate back to a completely normal life. Unless I developed so much burn from the radiation that I needed a break, in which case it would take longer.

Before you start radiation, they make you sign a contract-like agreement, committing yourself to showing up every day, to not taking any vacations without the doctor's permission. I suppose the contract ensures that people take radiation seriously, that they don't appear for appointments only willy-nilly, or suddenly decide to take that cruise to the Bahamas they've been planning for ten years, wrecking the treatment plan entirely. I can understand needing this statement of commitment for radiation. In my experience, radiation had no tangible, external effect, other than turning my skin progressively more alarming shades of red. I felt fine. So it would be easy to believe that missing a session here and there wouldn't hurt anything, because it was hard to believe it was actually having any effect.

But it was not the contract that got me there every day. It was the free cookies.

I'm a sucker for free food, plus I really love cookies. The radiation clinic had a tray of institutional-quality cookies in the reception area every day (yum yum), and you could have as many as you wanted. For Free. I was trying to lose the weight I'd put on during chemo (yes, counter-intuitively, given the nausea and all, you tend to gain weight during chemo because that's just how contrary chemo is), but one cookie a day fit into my diet. And they stocked all of my favorites: regular chocolate chip, chocolate with white chips, peanut butter, oatmeal-raisin. So at 2:40 p.m. every day, I would get into my car in St. Paul and head south towards home, where half-way in between, in Burnsville, just off the highway, I would stop for my free cookie. With a little dose of radiation on the side.

Why was this cookie important to me? Rediscovery of appetite? Some recompense for everything I'd been through? Proof that I was still in control because I could limit myself to one cookie? I don't know. I could have stopped at any Super America along the way and bought the same cookie for forty-nine cents. But I never did. And I never do now. It just doesn't taste the same.

The first step in the radiation process requires you to go in for a couple of hours so they can measure you, plaster cast you, and tattoo you. It's vital that the radiation blasts exactly the same area of your body every day, so you need to be in exactly the same position for each treatment, which is not that easy to achieve. During this preliminary exam and set-up appointment, the technician had me strip from the waist up (so last week by this time) then lie down on pretty much the coldest, hardest table I had yet encountered. I was also tended by pretty much the coldest, hardest technician I encountered in my two years of treatment, which may account for the coldness and hardness of the table. She seemed completely unsympathetic to my plight as I lay shivering and naked under the giant space-insect eye of the radiation machine, and she actually made me cry once a few weeks later. But I was tough, kind of, and could play along, at least most days.

After you lie down on the frigid table, they slide a giant beanbag-type plastic pillow under your head and shoulders and have you settle in, which feels like drowning naked in a box of packing pellets. Then they ask you to throw your arms up over your head, kind of like when the sun comes out to dry the rain off the itsy-bitsy spider, and nestle them down into the beanbag. By some magic of heat or chemicals, or witchy spell casting from the witchy technician, the beanbag then solidifies, memorializing this position, which you must assume at 3:26 p.m. every day for the next seven weeks.

The gallery of these plastic casts, stored in the shadows at the back of the radiation room, reminded me of the unfortunate souls who perished in the hot ash and lava of the erupting Mount Vesuvius, whose recast figures had been on display at the science museum a few years back. Arms thrown up around the head in a pointless final gesture of protection, because that's what our natures instruct us to do, regardless of the futility. My left arm gave me considerable pain in this position because I hadn't quite recovered the mobility I had lost the previous January, now a thousand years ago, when I broke my arm on the ice, and the problem had been compounded by the mastectomy. Enduring this daily pain provided another opportunity to think of the grandchildren I would meet one day. I'm doing this for you, kids.

Once they get you squared on the table, arms above your head in this position of pointless defensiveness, the space-insect eye emits a pale yellow rectangle of light, bisected by a grey X-Y axis, to frame your breast, or rather the area that used to include your breast. The rectangle is lined up to some mysterious specifications, and the technician tattoos small black dots at each end of the X axis, which defines the radiation field for subsequent treatments. I have those tattoos to this very day, although I hear you can ask your plastic surgeon to snip them out and stitch you up one more time. If you have the stamina for one more snipping and stitching session.

Finally, a couple hours later, you can lower your arms and put your supportive undergarment and sweater back on. They then set you up with a daily appointment time (3:20 p.m.) that will stay in your head forever, kind of like the exact times your kids were born, and you can be on your way. Don't forget to grab your free cookie on the way out.

I don't even like to imagine the radiation process and its attendant daily humiliations if you have anal cancer or vulvar cancer or testicular cancer or some other cancer located in a most awkward and intimate location. At least I'd been spared the spectacle of a plastic cast of my ass. Another reminder to count my blessings.

•　　•　　•　　•　　•

And so I began the seven weeks in which my day circled the vortex of 3:20 p.m. and my afternoon cookie. Same routine every day. Arrive at 3:18. Read the paper for a few minutes. Follow the technician back to an exam room. Strip from the waist up and don the pink and white hospital gown that never actually snapped in the back. Pad over to the radiation room, clutching the back of the gown. Sign the clipboard to prove I'd been there that day. Remove right side of body from gown and assume the position on the frigid treatment table, arms flung overhead into the plastic cast. Peer into the dim recesses of the cavernous, slightly ominous room, where massive, mysterious equipment lurked in the shadows. Close eyes and channel the peacefulness of the yoga studio, while the silent technician lined up the yellow light rectangle with my tattoos, then said, okay here we go, as she left the room. Lie really still, alone in the room, while the radiation machine thumped its menacing, rhythmic bass line for twelve seconds. Pull gown around chest, climb off the table, and head out the radiation room door toward the exam room, tossing out a half-hearted, see you tomorrow, to the technician on the way by, as she fiddled with the equipment panel but didn't bother to look up. Re-dress in the exam room. Grab cookie on the way out the door. Head home.

I saw the supervising doctor on Mondays, at least when she was there on Mondays, which was not always. Her job was basically to take a brief look at my chest and decide if the Crayola hue of my skin was closer to "Maine Lobster," which seemed to be an acceptable shade, or "Dirty Brick," which might be a reason to give me a day or two off. I'm sure she was a skilled practitioner who made good decisions about how much radiation to dose me with, and I'm sure her job involves many responsibilities that I am unaware of. But it seemed to me that this was the cushiest doctor job ever. At most, our interactions lasted two minutes. She never had to touch me or examine me in any way, other than to take a quick look when I pulled back my hospital gown to reveal the decorator shade of the day. Then she'd tell me to get some rest and drink plenty of fluids. See you next week.

After my twelve seconds of radiation every day, I would go home and slather aloe vera gel, the remedy of choice for crispy-burnt skin, on the rectangular red badge of courage that adorned my chest. You can buy aloe vera by the quart at the natural foods co-op, which of course you'll do because it's the thriftiest choice. Then you'll still have a pint or so left in the back of your bathroom cabinet for the next several years, buddying up to the constipation remedies. Just in case. Because you never know.

•   •   •   •   •

When I was about a week into radiation, I arrived at work one morning to hear that our faculty administrative assistant, Gloria, had been taken to the hospital the previous afternoon, after I departed for my radiation appointment, because she'd had some kind of alarming spell. It turned out that Gloria had a brain tumor. She had surgery in the next few days, then entered a daily radiation routine similar to mine.

Gloria returned to work pretty quickly, so we spent time comparing radiation notes. Her ordeal sounded worse than mine because keeping your head still and in the exactly the same position every day is more difficult that keeping your chest still and in exactly the same position every day. The radiation techs had made some sort of cage contraption for her head, the equivalent of my Pompeian-citizen arm-cast, and several times they had to stop the radiation treatment because she panicked with claustrophobia inside the contraption. But in general,

Gloria was a sunny, optimistic person who never said a bad word about anyone and was a joy to work with, so she never complained.

We finished our radiation treatments at about the same time in late March, and our colleagues threw us a radiation party, where everyone wore sunglasses and glow in the dark necklaces while we ate bagels, drank coffee, and talked about what we were doing for spring break.

But Gloria's tumor returned, was treated again, returned again, and was treated again. And about two years after her initial diagnosis, the tumor won. She was fifty-three.

Some of us make it out of the cancerland jungle, and some don't. There's no accounting for it, as far as I can tell. Why did I get breast cancer, which has pretty good odds of survival, instead of brain cancer, which does not? In the three years after I was diagnosed with cancer, I knew four people, three of them in my small town, plus Gloria, who died of brain cancer. And when I think about Gloria, I can't fathom that someone who was kind to me when I was first diagnosed, who sent me cards and flowers during my chemo, who asked after me every day, would herself succumb to this hateful disease while I survived it. She'd been healthy, and I had not. But then the tables had turned, for no apparent reason. I couldn't make sense of it. I still can't.

When I was first diagnosed, and was searching for a way to explain this calamity to myself and indulging my darker sense of humor, I joked about the plastic coating painted onto the concrete stairs in the corner stairwell of the law school in 2009. The plastic coating was meant, I think, to spruce things up and keep people like me from slipping. Like the coating you apply to your garage floor if you're obsessive-compulsive about a clean garage. It smelled terrible for several years, and in 2009, the noxious fumes filled the poorly ventilated stairwell. Every morning, as I descended those stairs to teach my class, I would think, these fumes are going to give me cancer. I really should take the other stairs.

Some might argue that thinking this thought every day gave me cancer. But there's no way to know if that could be true. And Gloria also had cancer. She probably didn't think that thought, because she was a better person than I am. So *could* it have been the stairway fumes? Is there a way to know, but we don't actually want to know?

Now I believe that simply inhabiting the world in the bodies we are given makes us susceptible to cancer. Cancer is an amoral proposition at the individual level. I don't think we cause it with our thoughts. But it's probably not an amoral proposition at the collective level. Collectively, we have agreed to expose ourselves to dangerous chemicals through our air, our water, our soil, because we desire a life that includes plastics, cars, cheap food, cheap energy—a vast inventory of modern-day accessories, or even necessities, that require chemicals and unnatural processes and toxic waste. We've agreed to take the risks, and some of us are the casualties.

I believe Gloria, and countless others, are these casualties. I'm just lucky that another miracle of modern life—chemotherapy—probably saved me.

•　　　•　　　•　　　•　　　•

I began the radiation slog, and it didn't take that long to get into the daily routine. Over the first few weeks, my rectangulate chest badge went from "June Morning in the Garden" pink to "Afternoon at the Beach" red to "Maine Lobster." But it didn't hurt, and I didn't suffer the fatigue or other side effects that some radiation patients do. The technicians continued to be on the cool to surly side, but hey, it was only ten minutes a day. Maybe their attitude was deliberately orchestrated to cool the burn.

So I was tooling along feeling good enough for a fun weekend, and we had a great one planned in early February. Friday night: dinner and cards at our house with three other couples, me cooking an elaborate meal for the first time post-diagnosis. Saturday night: larger dinner party, including many of my favorite people, at the home of our fabulous friends, Clara and Rob. Theme: Scandinavian Smorgasbord, including five kinds of herring from the last standing Scandinavian grocery store on Lake Street in Minneapolis, Pete's grandmother's Swedish Meatballs, Rob's fish stew, and homemade Aquavit—vodkas infused with various delightful flavors like horseradish and raspberry. Skol! I was in charge of the almond cake.

Friday afternoon after radiation, I stopped at the fancy suburban grocery to get a good piece of pork tenderloin, then headed home to cook. I put on a jazzy playlist—Ella Fitzgerald, Dave Brubeck, Mose Allison—and settled into a relaxed Friday afternoon of cooking, chatting with Elena, tossing scraps to Ruby, who keeps me company in the kitchen because I am a benevolent pack leader when it comes to food scraps, and sipping a glass of wine. Delicious smells filled the house. Elena switched on the fireplace.

Our guests arrived, and a lovely Friday evening ensued. We chatted through appetizers and a winter comfort food dinner of pork, mashed potatoes, and roasted vegetables, with plenty of laughs all around. But then I got up to clear the table for dessert.

During dinner, the chair next to mine had gotten snagged on the edge of the dining room rug, which had bunched up into a small hillock of rug. Rug, not water, was my hazard of choice this time. As I rose out of my seat and launched myself towards the kitchen, my foot caught on the hillock of rug. I fell.

I didn't fall far. Just a slight down, and no crack. I caught myself on a nearby counter, so really it was just a sudden forward propulsion of my torso, stopped short when my hands caught the first available surface. In fact, my hands were the only part of my upper body that contacted any surface.

Oops, I laughed. Clumsy me, I said, as I righted myself and took a few more steps towards the kitchen. Then I realized that blood was pouring down my chest.

It was February, and we live in Minnesota, so I was wearing my winter uniform: a supportive undergarment, a camisole, a long sleeved shirt, a sweater, and maybe even a fleece jacket over that. So I was the only one aware of the blood. I grabbed Jeff's arm as he rinsed dishes at the kitchen sink and whispered in his ear, come upstairs with me.

When I put it that way, it sounds a little racy. Did he think I was inviting him upstairs for a quickie? Did he think I was losing my mind? And I'm not sure what our guests thought when both hosts suddenly disappeared up the stairs. Valentine surprise for someone? Large gifts all around, hidden in the upstairs closet?

I got to our bathroom, where I rooted through layers of clothing to locate the source of the bleeding. When I finally made my way down to the core, I discovered that the original mastectomy incision on my right side, the one Dr. Smith had partially re-stitched in December, had split wide open like an overripe summer fruit, exposing the pearly sheet of corpse-derma tissue to the open air.

It was a clean split, leaving behind a grinning orifice, like a cheap zipper broken open through the middle but with both ends intact. The edges of the incision were smooth, lip-like, as if they had never been stitched together at all. After I sopped up the initial spill of blood with a towel, I found that the area was not bleeding much at all. Just seeping a bit around the edges. A pupil-less, alien eye stared from my chest.

Jeff and I huddled in the bathroom for a few minutes, somehow thinking we could manage this on our own. But clearly not. My insides were exposed to the world, and we soon realized that Band-Aids would not remedy the situation. So Jeff looked up Dr. Smith's phone number, called the answering service, and left a message. I felt no pain, my internal parts seemed to be staying snugly in place under the sheath of corpse-derma, and the bleeding remained minimal. I didn't think I needed to go to the local emergency room, where they would probably have no idea what to do with me anyway.

One of Dr. Smith's partners, Dr. Larson, called me back a few minutes later and listened as I described what had happened.

Huh, she said. That's not good. Just goes to show that radiation and reconstruction don't mix.

Thanks for that feedback, I thought.

Yeah, I said. That's what Dr. Smith told me. I wouldn't have chosen this course had we known I needed radiation.

I looked down at the alien eye and mopped up a little blood starting to ooze out the corners. Jeff hovered outside the bathroom, not sure whether our guests or I needed him more. Thank goodness Elena wasn't home.

After Dr. Larson assessed how much I was bleeding and whether I was in pain, she agreed that I should not go to the local emergency room.

They might not have the expertise to respond to this the way we would want them to, she said. I'll call the hospital up here and see if we can get a surgery suite for the morning. Put some gauze on the area and call me if anything changes. Don't eat or drink after midnight.

I sent Jeff downstairs to check on our guests, then sat down on the commode. I put my head in my hands and cried for a minute, dreading the thought of another surgery the next morning. But bending over only made the bleeding worse. So I pulled myself together, patched things up as best I could, reinstalled my layers of clothing, and went downstairs.

As with many cancer-imposed situations, life's usual playbook does not prepare you for this dinner party. Instead, you need one of those novelty quiz books stacked next to the checkout at the bookstore, meant to tempt the impulse shopper. Worst Case Hypothetical: Your chest splits open during a dinner party at your home, and you notice that you have begun to bleed profusely. What do you do? What should your guests do? Discuss.

Downstairs, Jeff had outlined the basic facts to our guests, who were all long-time friends of ours with a variety of medical problems themselves. He figured they could cope. As I entered the dining room, a chorus of dear, sympathetic faces turned towards me, wondering what would happen next.

So, I said, wiping away my tears. Let's play cards.

And we did. Because what else are you going to do?

•   •   •   •   •

The next morning, Jeff drove me to the suburban hospital where Dr. Larson was on duty for the weekend. It's quiet in the surgery department on Saturdays. Not much happens that can't wait until Monday, I suppose, especially first thing in the morning. After an intake interview, a nurse wheeled me through a deserted corridor to the day-surgery unit and handed me over to another nurse in the surgery prep suite.

On days like this, you can't predict what will stay with you, easing your way on the cancer road. Today, it was the nurse in the surgery prep suite. I told him about my recurring trouble with IVs, so he went and got a pile of warm blankets to swaddle my arm and coax the veins to the surface. He also had me drink a big glass of water, then relax under the blankets for ten minutes before he even tried to insert the IV. Minutes later, the IV slid into my arm on the first try.

Take that, arrogant hospital anesthesiologist.

I note this here for a reason. Based on this simple act of kindness and care, which maybe this nurse could afford because it was Saturday morning and not much was happening in the day-surgery world, the following summer I chose this hospital, over my original mastectomy hospital, for the major surgery occasioned by this reconstruction failure. That turned out to be a questionable decision. I'll get to that part of the story later. But it just shows how a little bit of compassion makes a huge difference to a person in distress, and that compassion carries forward in ways you may not expect.

Dr. Larson came in to take a look, just to make sure the expander implant couldn't be salvaged. When I opened my gown and pointed the unblinking alien eye in her direction, she grimaced.

Ouch, she said. Okay, see you in the surgery suite.

Wait, I said. What's it going to look like when you're done?

I'd lain awake for a while the night before, worrying about this. Would it be a nice, flat expanse, a blank slate? Or would it be an alien landscape, spawn of the alien eye?

Well, the expander has to come out, she said, and I can't put in a new one because of the radiation. And I'll need to put in a drain on that side, which can come out in a few weeks. You'll have to wait at least six months after radiation ends before you try reconstruction again. You can talk to Dr. Smith about it in the office next week. You'll need about a week off from radiation, but then you can start up your treatments again. In the meantime, it will just look—well, stitched up.

I lay back and shut my eyes, not wanting to think about what that meant and dismayed by this further delay. At this rate, I wouldn't be done with reconstruction for another year. Hadn't I paid my cancer dues by now?

But I didn't have much time to think. Soon, the double doors opened for me once again. And once again, I lay on my back in the surgical suite and counted backward from one hundred until I was gone.

In recovery a couple hours later, I kept losing the consciousness thread and slipping back into the comforting darkness of sleep, or something like it. But for reasons I didn't understand, the recovery room nurse was on a mission to get me moving, and she insisted I sit up and try to shake it off. I resisted, she insisted. I resisted, she insisted. I wondered if she had a party to get to or if they could all go home early if only I cooperated. Then I remembered that *we* had a party to get to, and I was in charge of the almond cake. So I swung my legs over the side of the bed and, through the fog, began to pull on my clothes while the nurse read me discharge instructions and Jeff went to get the car. My chest was once again completely wrapped in gauze. I would not have to confront this new reality for a day or two.

I slept in the car, and Jeff settled me into bed when we got home, where I slept several more hours. I woke up around six o'clock, about when the Scandinavian dinner party was scheduled to start, and decided with Jeff, what the heck. My friends will still love me even if I don't bring the almond cake, and it's only four blocks away, so I can come home any time. Let's go to the party.

So we went to the party, where I ate herring for the first time ever. Yum. The meatballs and fish stew were also delicious. We skipped dessert, but made up for it with multiple rounds of Aquavit, which I did not mix with pain medication. Despite my distaste for pithy, optimistic aphorisms, another one proved true: Laughter *is* the best medicine. Skol.

•　　•　　•　　•　　•

On Monday morning, I wanted to shower. So I stood in the bathroom and carefully unwound the gauze that had swaddled my chest for two days, holding my breath as I got closer and closer to ground zero.

And indeed, it was horrifying. Against the palate of Maine Lobster, my skin was bruised and puffy. Where there had been a C-cup foothill, there was now Deadman's Gulch—a violent, uneven, pinched and tucked gash across the flattened right side of my chest. Dr. Larson had preserved the skin that had covered the foothill, but had pulled it together across the middle like a drawstring bag, pleating here and stitching there to bind together the edges that had been torn asunder.

"Hideous" came to mind. A word I had never before applied to myself. I took a deep breath, tore my eyes away from the mirror, and got in the shower.

The next morning, I went to see Dr. Smith for follow up and to discuss my options. He shook his head about mixing radiation and reconstruction, and he reminded me that the important thing was to make sure I was cancer free.

Yeah, yeah, I thought. Tell me something I don't know.

The reconstruction would have to wait, he said. If all went well from here, we could start talking again in June. But the good news was, I could still have reconstruction on that side. It would just be more complicated and would probably involve the "lat flap" procedure, where he would take tissue from my back and install it on my front.

More surgery, I thought, as I followed Ashley to the photo room.

I could have considered calling the whole thing off at that point. But I didn't. I felt ugly, deformed, and I was desperate for it to be right again. I knew normal was not possible—I was long past normal when it came to my chest. But I believed Dr. Smith would do his best to at least make me feel as normal as possible, whatever that meant.

After a photo op with Ashley, I left the office and went down the block, where I had discovered a more conveniently located mastectomy products shop. There, courtesy of Blue Cross, I obtained a C-cup prosthesis and a couple new supportive undergarments to hold it in place. I opted for the temporary, fiberfill prosthesis, later nicknamed Booby the Breast—not quite a Beanie Baby, but close—rather than the more permanent silicone prosthesis, because temporary seemed like the more hopeful choice. Once I installed Booby under my Minnesota winter uniform, you would never guess what I'd been through in the last few days.

My prosthesis now lives in a box on the top shelf of my closet, nestled into the dark next to my wig and my mastectomy bras. I hear that Booby the Breast is going to be worth a lot of money someday. Maybe more than Seymour the Seal. If only I'd kept the tag.

•　　•　　•　　•　　•

A week later, I resumed the radiation routine. The routine went smoothly overall. But on a Tuesday late in February, I had a day that brought home how vulnerable I still felt, and how much cancer still controlled my life.

In the morning, I saw Dr. Chen for a chemotherapy follow-up appointment. At the appointment, I learned that Bonnie was moving to a different clinic, and I was introduced to her replacement. Her replacement, Sue, was pleasant enough, but not particularly my type. She was older and didn't really look me in the eye or seem to care much about whether I was safe at home. I didn't want to have coffee with her, and I doubted her grasp of constipation remedies.

As Sue checked my vitals and charted my answers, I realized just how deeply I had bonded with Bonnie, the one constant through this whole process who had never let me down. Sure, Dr. Smith was great, but he hadn't warned me about the possible radiation mishap, had he? Bonnie was there whenever I called for help in my most miserable moments, and she always had the right answer. I realized I might never see Bonnie again because you're not actually supposed to be friends with your medical professionals. The rules of professionalism say you can't exchange emails or phone numbers or make plans for coffee next week. I could barely hold back my tears.

After my exam, I sat for an hour waiting to be called to the desk to make an appointment, the appointment clerk inexplicably delayed. I mourned Bonnie the whole time. I'd had to wait before, but not like this, and outrage just added to my catalogue of hurts. I was, after all, a working girl and didn't have time to waste sitting around the oncologist's office.

Appointment finally made, I went to work for a few hours and fumed in my office. Then at the usual 2:40, I left my office to drive to my radiation appointment. I arrived at 3:18, two minutes ahead of schedule, but then sat for another hour in *that* waiting room, resisting the cookie tray, with no explanation about the delay. When the witchy technician finally called me back, we got right down to the business of clothes off and equipment fiddling and arms overhead, which now exposed the hideous, mutilated gulch to scrutiny every day. When the technician disappeared, I was left in that position on the cold table, alone, ungowned, no explanation, for about ten minutes.

I didn't spend a lot of time feeling sorry for myself during my cancer ordeal, but this sequence of abandonments left me bereft. Tears again began to slide down my cheeks and into my ears. I lay there, unable to muster the nerve to grab my gown and storm out. I was alone on my back in the vast universe, and no one seemed to care. I always knew I was completely on my own, and here! Here was the proof! I was paralyzed, unable to draw on the treasure trove of love and support I'd been blessed with in the previous six months, although I knew in my head it was there, ready to comfort me in every moment.

The radiation technician finally reappeared, told me they were ready, and headed out of the room. Next came the twelve seconds of boom boom boom, followed by silence. I was off the table before the reverberations stopped. As I passed the technician on the way out, she actually looked up and noticed my mascara-stained face.

Oh, she said. Are you upset? You're so easy. You're never any trouble. You never move!

Her reaction fed my despair. This was not about whether I was any trouble for her. This was not about whether I could lay still long enough to make her job easy. I blew past her to the changing room, yanked on my clothes, and stormed out, ignoring even the cookies on my way past the desk.

When I got home, I poured out the day to Jeff as he sat at the kitchen island, ignoring the stack of ungraded assignments in front of him. He got up to make me some tea, and the dog moved from her place under the dining room table to her place in the kitchen, next to my feet. Gradually, as the account of my day tumbled out, I wound down. When I got out the potatoes to start dinner, Jeff took them away, then took out his phone and ordered pizza. Elena came home and gave me a hug, and I could once again feel the care that I'd lost touch with during the day.

I didn't want to go back to radiation the next day, or the next. I thought about going shopping instead. How, instead of taking a right on Nicollet Avenue when I got off the highway, I could take a left into the mall parking lot. Then I could stroll through the vast, climate-controlled anonymity that is Macy's, where I would chat with the nice clerks, who would want to know if I was having a great day. I could indulge in the addictive comforts of American consumerism. Maybe drink a nice latte at Starbucks and try on some shoes.

But I didn't do that. I continued to turn right onto Nicollet Avenue every day, into the vast medical complex, eyes on the baked-goods prize.

• • • • •

The following week, tentacles of red began to radiate out from the scar on the *left* side of my chest, the un-radiated, reconstruction-intact side. Just testing the waters, like an octopus from behind its rock. For once, I was glad that the radiation doctor was available on Monday to take a look. She poked and prodded a bit, then decided I should probably see Dr. Smith, just to check it out. So the next day, I found myself once again on Dr. Smith's exam table, looking at the door over my left shoulder, while *he* poked and prodded. He announced that he wanted to re-incise the scar, stitch me up again, and put me on two weeks of antibiotics.

Two weeks later, the new incision wasn't healing well, so he cut me open another time, stitched me up again, and handed me another prescription. I think we may have gone through this routine three times in all during February and March.

But at this point, what did it matter? Hideous on one side, unsightly on the other. I was getting used to the wreck that was my new body, and I wondered if I would ever emerge on the other side.

Chapter Eighteen

All of a sudden, at the beginning of April, everything cleared.

I had taken another break from radiation in early March, partly because my chest was trending towards a "Barbequed Chicken Forgotten on the Grill" hue, and partly because, defying the radiation contract, I wanted to visit my best friend from high school, Pat, in Seattle for a few days. Pat likes to spend money and has plenty to spend, and it's always fun to relax and catch up at her beautiful house across Puget Sound for a couple days, then blow a night or two riding around Seattle in a chauffeured town car in search of the best martinis and chocolate cake. Just what the doctor ordered.

So radiation stretched out until the end of March, but was wrapped up nicely with the glow-in-the-dark party at work. My chemo port had come out in January, which was an optimistic choice (some doctors wait a year, just to make sure), and my left-side incision seemed to be healing, finally, after several cut and stitch sessions. I was advised to take a daily dose of Tamoxifen for five years, a drug that shuts down estrogen production, but was otherwise done with Dr. Chen. Dr. Smith didn't want to see me again until June.

Oh, the freedom.

For eight months, I had not gone more than a week without being examined, biopsied, prodded, cut open, poisoned, irradiated, scanned, or medicated in some way. Cancer treatment takes over your life, and you just get sick of it. It defines your day and your week. It dictates how you sleep, what you eat, whether you can tolerate a drink or not, how well your bodily functions perform, whether you feel like going out to the pub with your friends. But now, in the month most focused on renewal and rebirth, cruel or not, the window opened, and fresh air filled the room. I didn't see a doctor for almost six weeks.

My 6:30 a.m. walk with Ruby was noticeably brighter every morning as spring unfolded. The lilacs bloomed, filling the air with their heavy perfume, the grass turned to green velvet, and the cardinals said pretty, pretty, pretty as we walked by. And I believed that it was so.

And, in that first week of April, my hair began to grow back—a true sign of spring. After a week of sprouting stubble, I put the wig away in the closet and went to work au naturelle. I was meeting individually with students that week, and I felt compelled to apologize to everyone who entered my office, afraid I might shock them with my just-shorn look. But they took it in stride, and pretty soon I could pretend that I had this "haircut" by choice.

When you choose to go out in public with this haircut, you have to be prepared for variations on the Having Cancer in Public problem. Sporting obvious post-chemo hair, I encountered both stranger sympathy and survivor networking. Where else but in Target, of course, which is really our twenty-first-century public square, because who doesn't go there at least once a week?

I was looking for light bulbs in the hardware section when a man I didn't know caught my eye and said, I like your haircut. Which was clearly code for, let's talk about cancer. I tried to escape, but to no avail. I ended up cornered in aisle seventeen for about twenty minutes, hearing about his own cancer ordeal. I only escaped when I accepted one of those plastic wristbands made popular by Lance Armstrong, imprinted with this fellow's Cancer Survival website address. I appreciated the thought, but dropped the wristband in the trashcan on my way out.

Other people would stop to tell me how great my hair was going to be when it grew back in. Maybe red, or curly, or red *and* curly—certainly, they seemed to promise, there would be a new me, ready for a new life, that would emerge from this ugly duckling stage. Again, I appreciated the support and the good intentions. But often these were inane conversations, during which I would nod and smile, eager to get back to my shopping list. Because, for godsakes, I just wanted to be away from cancer for a while. Can I please get back to my life now? I wanted to say. But it's hard to say that to complete strangers, or even friends, who want to be helpful.

About mid-May, Samantha gave me my first real, post-chemo haircut, so my hair actually had a shape to it, which signaled a return to real life. In fact, my hair came in salt-and-pepper grey, the same way it went out, with maybe a new, slight cowlick on the left temple. My body hair also returned on schedule, although for a couple of weeks, my skin felt like I had goosebumps all the time. This was just the individual hairs, newly emerging from the follicles, but it was odd and disconcerting to be so bumpy after the months of smooth, lovely skin.

Because of Bonnie's departure, and because I never bonded with Dr. Chen, I decided to switch oncologists for my follow-up care. In May, I had my first three-month oncology check up with my new oncologist, Dr. McCarthy. Dr. McCarthy was a kindly, slightly eccentric older lady who wore green tennis shoes and took in pets that belonged to cancer patients who could no longer care for them. At the time, I think she had something like thirty dogs and fifty cats, not to mention the birds and exotics. I don't know how she took care of them. But I completely approved of this use of *her* doctor money. She was the church lady of the oncology clinic. I imagined she might hand me a casserole on my way out of the clinic.

Also, Bonnie! Dr. McCarthy saw patients at a different clinic than Dr. Chen, and it happened to be the clinic Bonnie had transferred to. So during my first appointment at the new clinic, Bonnie tracked me down, and we spent a good fifteen minutes catching up. I tried not to feel guilty about her other patients, who were probably waiting alone, shivering in their pink gowns down the hall.

Dr. McCarthy came in to review my history, and as I chronicled my increasingly complicated story, I could not prevent a few tears from welling up in the corners of my eyes. For the rest of the appointment, between the pokings and proddings, she spent her time alternating between hugging me and assuring me that I was going to be fine, just fine. Hug. Fine, dear, fine. Take a deep breath for me. Okay. You're going to be fine. Breathe normally. Hug, hug. Raise your arms. Fine, just fine. Lower your arms. Fine. I know you're going to be fine. You can sit up. Hug. Hug.

And I was fine. Great, in fact. I had cleared my first post-cancer check-up. I had a hairstyle, of sorts. It was May, and the expanse of summer rolled out in front of me. To celebrate, I stopped at my favorite bakery on the way home and got a high-end, expensive cookie and a latte. Then I settled in to enjoy this new game: a doctor free, cancer-free life. At least for a while.

•   •   •   •   •

Between mid-May and mid-July, I did live a relatively doctor-free, cancer-free life. I had a colonoscopy, which had been due the previous summer, but was delayed when I entered the breast cancer spanking machine. But that felt somewhat—ah—cleansing, frankly. And at our house, you don't complain about colonoscopies, because Sam has had more colonoscopies in his short life than Jeff and I will ever have in ours, put together. For Sam, colonoscopies are akin to getting your teeth cleaned. A couple times a year whether you need it or not.

Then Elena, who had been through so much this year, graduated from high school on a perfectly brilliant June afternoon. I felt blessed to be there, and I camouflaged my tears behind sunglasses all afternoon. I had made it to this first big, post-cancer milestone, and I was ecstatic—for me and for her. During the ceremony, as Elena received her diploma, two bald eagles circled overhead, which I believed were sent just for us.

In early June, I saw Dr. Smith so he could gauge whether I might be ready for my re-reconstruction surgery at the end of July. If so, and if all went well, I would be ready to return to work when classes began again the third week of August. Then when classes ended in December, I could have the new expander, which would be placed during the July surgery, removed and replaced with the permanent implant.

I felt good about this schedule. I would be essentially done with reconstruction a year later than I originally planned, but the urgency had worn off over the last six months. And remember: goals make me happy, and this gave me a new set of goals. Dr. Smith agreed to put me on the surgery schedule for July 22, with the proviso that in mid-July, he could change his mind if he didn't think I was ready.

And mostly, during this time, I let my anxiety about recurrence go. In fact, I even felt a slightly shameful but invigorating sense of relief that I'd finally had "my" cancer experience. I'd secretly worried about cancer for years—the horrible near-death disease, the chemotherapy, the struggle to maintain the will to live. But this had already happened to me. I'd done okay, and here I was on the other side. I shouldn't have to do it again, and even if I did, I knew I could handle it. So I could jump into the next stage of my life free of the dark expectation that I would at some point have cancer, which had followed me around like a noxious shade for years, for no rational reason.

During these couple of months, I continued my gratitude practice on my morning walks, and I listened several times a day to the Talking Heads song, *Once in a Lifetime*. I think that song means different things to different people, and the Stop Making Sense album version (aka, the RIGHT version) sends a completely different message than the Remain in Light album version (aka, the WRONG version). To me, the song captures this sense of distance I sometimes feel from what has actually happened in my life (*Well, how did I get here?*) and reminds me to not let convention, expectation, and anxiety run things. (*This is not my beautiful house. This is not my beautiful wife.*) Rather, I should ride the wave of each individual day, own my own life, and enjoy what comes my way. (*Letting the days go by. Letting the days go by.*) Such is the power of a good tune.

In June, fueled by my "one more day" mantra and my obsessive repetition of this song, I decided to throw financial caution to the wind and plan a trip to London with Elena. A post-graduation treat for her and a post-cancer treat for me. I also bought a fantastic, slightly risky dress to wear to her graduation party. And I bought my first new car ever, a brand new Ford Fiesta, to take me forward into the next phase of life. The car had a great sound system, a sunroof, interior mood lighting in six selectable colors, and leather seats, with a magenta exterior. My friend Rob, a poet, called it the lipstick car.

I suppose you could see these indulgences as motivated by a predictable post-cancer attitude: taking-life-by-storm-because-I-know-I'm-going-to-die. I like to believe that I approached life with the same live-to-the-max attitude before cancer. But I did feel a renewed energy, a willingness to take more risks, a visceral realization that worrying about cramped resources and unlikely consequences would only impoverish my life. It was like I finally got the equation the right way around. You don't embrace life and live to the fullest—travel; acquire things you love and shed the things you don't; make that slightly risky move—because you know you're going to die. You do those things because you know you're going to live.

So I got into my new Fiesta, turned up *Once in a Lifetime* on the kickass sound system, chose an interior lighting color to suit my mood, and accelerated into the future.

• • • • •

The week before Elena and I were to leave for London, two rough, red, blotchy spots appeared on the right side of my chest, near Deadman's Gulch, each about the size of a nickel. I went in to see the nurse practitioner who works with Dr. McCarthy, and we debated whether they could be tick bites or, on the other hand, cancer. She prescribed a course of antibiotics to cover the tick bite theory, and we agreed to wait to see if they went away.

And so I entered into my first cancer recurrence anxiety cycle, which has happened probably half a dozen times since then and has thus become commonplace. The cycle goes like this. You have something slightly unusual happening in your body—a funny lump, swollen glands for no reason, a blotchy spot, a backache, a non-viral cough—that in your pre-cancer days, would maybe have triggered the thought, hmm, I wonder if that could be cancer. In the pre-cancer days, you would then apply some ice or take some Tylenol, and wait a few hours or a few days, and it would go away, entirely forgotten. Instead, you now call your oncologist, they bring you in, you negotiate how much investigation they think appropriate and how much you want to put up with, you submit to that investigation, and then you wait over the weekend to find out if it's cancer or not. Given your history, it's plausible that it could be. Chances are, it's not.

Ten days later, in our London hotel room, red buses lumbering by outside the window, I decided the blotches were not going away and were perhaps getting worse. So I emailed Jeff, who got in touch with Dr. McCarthy's office, who got in touch with Dr. Smith's office, who set up a biopsy appointment a few days after I got home. I needed to see Dr. Smith anyway, to confirm that we could go ahead with the July surgery, and it would make no sense to embark on major reconstruction surgery the next week if my cancer was back. Elena and I were having a wonderful trip, every day a perfect London day, and I managed to not think about cancer too much. But I was glad to have a plan for my return.

On Tuesday, a week before my scheduled surgery, I saw Dr. Smith, and he once again cut out a little chunk here and a little chunk there, stitched me up, and sent me on my way. I held my breath as I looked over his full head of hair, at my left shoulder, towards the door, but he did not say that I was not ready for surgery. And while he thought the biopsy was prudent, he didn't seem worried about the results. See you next week, he said, as he left the exam room.

•   •   •   •   •

The night before surgery, I went to yoga, thinking my body would be more prepared for surgery the next day if I went into it with a yogic mindset. The class that night was taught by James, everybody's favorite gay yoga teacher. James is the kind of yogi who can put his feet behind his neck and can then probably walk across the room on his hipbones, all the while giving you helpful advice about how to improve your own posture. James left the studio a few years ago, and it will never be the same without him.

Anyway, I was chatting with James as I racked my mat and put on my shoes, and I mentioned that I wouldn't be in class for several weeks because I was having major surgery. I think he knew that I'd been through breast cancer treatment the year before because it was pretty hard to miss my perennially hatted head during yoga. Besides, Amy, the owner of the studio is extremely generous and community-minded, and she gives anyone going through cancer treatment six months of free yoga, a gift she had extended to me earlier in the year.

I proceeded to tell James all the exciting details about how they were going to take a chunk of skin and muscle from my back and migrate it through my body, underneath the skin of my armpit, with blood supply intact, then pop it out the front and fill it with an expander to create a new boob on my right side.

Although James is a wonderful guy and an outstanding yoga teacher, the expression on his face showed just how much he really didn't want to know all that. Or maybe any of it. Not the slightest bit. And once it was out of my mouth, I couldn't take it back.

During cancer treatment, I guess you get used to strong emotions and physical details being commonplace, and your filter gets a little bit broken. At least mine did. I think back about my neighbor Laurie, my hair stylist Samantha, James—I'm sure there were others I dumped information on because I needed to tell someone, and there they were. I would do that differently now. I would be more thoughtful about who wanted to hear my story in the moment and who did not. You never know what your story may trigger in someone else, and I wish I'd had better sense about respecting that.

I can't take any of it back. But I can learn to forgive myself for the mistakes I made during cancer. I can learn to let go of this past, and assume the best about the people around me—that they have forgiven my mistakes too.

• • • • •

The next morning, Jeff and I headed west through the emerald July cornfields towards the highway, recreating the many trips down the same road the previous summer. But this summer, the road construction was completed, the sun was shining brightly, and we were headed to the destination by choice, sort of, rather than necessity. I had chosen to have this surgery at the big suburban hospital connected to Dr. Smith's office by a skyway, rather than the downtown hospital where I'd had my mastectomy. Partly because of the nice nurse in February, who knew how to get an IV going in a compassionate way. Partly because it was near my favorite bakery, so Jeff could easily bring me treats (Peanut butter chocolate chip cookies! Almond croissants!) during my four-day stay. And partly because, earlier that year, the downtown hospital had weathered a highly publicized scandal involving a nurse stealing pain killers from surgery patients, leaving them to endure excruciating procedures with insufficient medication. Ouch. The suburban hospital was also a little closer to home.

This time, I had no doubts. The biopsy from the previous week had come back clean. So I walked boldly into the surgery prep area, stood at attention with good humor while Dr. Smith mapped out his plan on my chest and my back with his Sharpie marker, and smiled and waved at Jeff as they wheeled me through the double doors into the OR area.

And Dr. Ryan had been right. His colleagues over in plastics really were doing some amazing work. It took about four hours for Dr. Smith to carve out a football-shaped piece of skin and tissue from my mid-back, including part of my latissimus-dorsi muscle, migrate the whole business, with the blood vessels intact, *through* my body, open up Deadman's Gulch on the front, stitch the football into the Gulch, place an expander in the resulting pocket, and sew me up, back and front. When Jeff wrote an email to my friends and family that night, he described the surgery as Dr. Smith playing with tinker toys—just put the pieces together in any fashion you want, to make an exciting new whole. In fact, later, to combat hospital boredom, I spent some time on the Internet checking out the deep credentials of the various doctors I had visited in the past year, and I discovered that Dr. Smith actually has an engineering degree from a prestigious university. Which made total sense, given the tinker toy nature of his work. And if you can't decide between engineering and medicine, do both! What a happy result: make more doctor money than anybody else! Okay, *and* help people feel whole and live better lives. Let's not forget that part.

Once again, I came around with a drain in my chest and, this time, one in my back. But the surgery had been short enough that I did not need a catheter, although I did have the inflatable booties to keep my blood pumping back up the pipes. Dr. Smith had warned me that the recovery from this surgery might be longer than the mastectomy recovery, and I would definitely need at least three days in the hospital, probably four. But this surgery seemed much easier to me. Maybe because I felt in control and not afraid. Maybe because I knew I would be ready to return to work in a few weeks, with little time lost. And maybe because this was the end of the ordeal, not the beginning.

This hospital had mostly shared patient rooms, and I came out of my fog in the middle of my first night to realize that the commotion meant I was getting a roommate. The nurses left the curtain between us drawn, which then seemed a bit awkward in the morning. We were literally lying there about four feet apart, but we had no rulebook telling us how to start an acquaintance under these circumstances. Neither one of us could get out of bed without assistance, and although I could have reached the curtain, just flinging it open seemed rude and possibly painful. So I lay there for a couple hours wondering if she preferred Home and Garden TV or the Food Network, or if I should just stay plugged into my iPod listening to *Once in a Lifetime* and Copland's *Billy the Kid*.

She was clearly the braver person because she finally said something to me, and I responded politely, and then we had the freshman week conversation. Which is probably the same conversation you have when you go to prison, although I don't know that for sure since I have not had that experience.

Where are you from? What are you in for (aka what's your major)? When do you get sprung/graduate? Any family around? What's the food like around here?

Jeanie turned out to be a politically liberal person from a politically conservative town, where she worked for the school district, which was in deep shit for various shenanigans involving uncontrolled bullying. So we got along just fine. We liked the same books and had similar doubts about the feminist cred of *What Not to Wear*, even though we loved the show, which was on at noon, and she kept me entertained with all the details about the school district story that had not made it into the papers. I was sorry to see her go on the morning of day three. The time passed like a breeze.

I had a nagging feeling that the staff at this hospital was not as competent as the staff at the downtown hospital, which I found disappointing, considering the competence of the February day-surgery nurse. But their procedures seemed sloppy. The nursing assistants would sometimes not bother to check my wristband when they came to record the volume of pee I'd managed to produce or to check my vitals. Or the pee would sit in the pee collector in the bathroom for hours, until I finally dumped it myself. Or they would give me medication and not follow up on whether I had taken it. Or they would neglect the little things, like whether I needed water or was getting out of bed enough and walking around. I find the obsessive wristband checking annoying, like everyone else, but I see the necessity. And having spent a lot of time in hospitals with Sam in the past few years, not to mention my own experiences, I knew the protocols. Here, I found them lacking.

Nonetheless, I healed quickly and was ready to go home on the morning of day four. Just a few more weeks and the drains could come out. I was on the home stretch.

Chapter Nineteen

Of course, you really shouldn't think thoughts like: Now I am on the Home Stretch. You totally jinx it, even if you don't believe in stuff like that. Like when it occurs to you in the shower one morning that you have not had a cold in ages, and then by dinnertime, whammo, your throat is sore and your sinuses are starting to fill up. I do not yet know if you cause the cold by thinking the shower-thought, or if your body actually intuitively knows you are getting the cold, even though your brain has not caught on yet, and that knowledge triggers the thought itself. I'm hoping to have an answer to this question within my lifetime. And I hope the answer is the former, so I can then work on figuring out how to avoid the shower thought in the first place, thereby curing the common cold.

I know. Good luck with that.

I spent the next two weeks lying on the couch healing. It was late July and early August, when life pretty much comes to a stop in a small academic town, so I wasn't missing much. Carolyn corralled the casserole ranks, and people brought us food and stopped by to visit. Elena went out to weed at the organic farm and returned home with bags of just-picked vegetables, which delivered vitamin-packed, healing goodness with just a deep inhale. Sweet corn season started again, and I partook with gusto and gratitude. I was ready to move on.

About two weeks after the surgery, I saw Dr. Smith for a post-surgical check-up. He pronounced that everything looked good and I should come back next week, when he would remove the drains and begin the Growing-Up-Skipper expansion process again. I had two drains, one in front and one in back, and had endured the usual drain stripping and fluid measuring ritual for the past two weeks, and I was tired of it. With one drain in back and one in front, I couldn't find a comfortable sleeping position. Also, summer clothes don't accommodate surgical drains nearly as handily as fall and winter clothes. And being saddled with drains just did not suit my mood of cancer-free optimism.

Can't you *please* take them out? I pleaded. I really don't want to wait another week. There's really not that much drainage.

I tried making sad eyes at him, but I've always been much better at logic than at feminine wiles, even when the situation involves a handsome man.

I'm sleeping really badly because of the drains, I said. If I sleep better, surely I will heal faster?

This is the one moment in Dr. Smith's treatment of me when I think he made the wrong decision. He probably should not have relented. He clearly was reluctant. But I guess my stellar logic and persuasion skills overwhelmed his good judgment. Or maybe my lawyer status had made him nervous all along.

Hmm. Okay. He hesitated. Well, I guess we could do it today. He reached for the gloves and the gauze. Soon, with a one, two, three, schloop, they were out. What a relief.

Dr. Smith applied a patch of gauze and some tape. While he worked, and I admired his ability to never get drain tube gloop on his expensive suits, he told me to remember to take it easy. I was still not far out from surgery and needed to let myself recover.

Okay, I thought. Whatever. I'm almost done.

I slept well on Tuesday night, and Wednesday was great: drain-free and forward-looking. I almost felt back to normal. Thursday morning, I got up a little late since Jeff was still walking Ruby until my back healed completely and I could handle the sled-dog-on-a-leash routine. I got in the shower and let the hot water envelop me, drains and lanyard free for the first time in two weeks.

As the hot water poured down, I started to realize that I wasn't actually feeling that great, but couldn't quite pinpoint why. Maybe I'd overdone it the previous day because I was so relieved to be restored to an unencumbered body. Maybe the water was a little too hot for August. Besides, I'd had major surgery only two weeks before. I was probably pushing myself a little too hard on my quest for normal. I should follow my doctor's advice and take it easy.

But in a few minutes, a wave of weakness and dizziness overcame me. I stepped out of the shower without drying off, pulled my terry robe around me, as I had done when I was too wrung out from chemo to dry off, and sat down on the commode. I put my head between my knees for a few minutes, then got up, washed down a few Tylenol with a glass of water, and decided to go back to bed since I had nothing pressing to do that day. I chalked it up to too much activity the day before, coupled with too much steam and heat on a warm August day.

I slept most of the morning, felt better, had some lunch, and then slept some more. I didn't feel terrible, but I didn't feel as well as I had felt the past couple of days. Maybe it was just the predictable ups and downs of the recovery process, I thought. I will probably be fine tomorrow.

Although I am generally so compliant and on top of medical issues, it did not occur to me until after dinner, when I started feeling really not well at all, to take my temperature. I never run a fever. My holding temperature seems to be about 97.1, like a Lite FM radio station, which probably reflects my temperament as well. I'm not quite down the dial to laconic NPR news, but I'm nowhere near the energetic classic rock and hip-hop in the dial's upper reaches. In the past twenty years, I've probably only run a fever above 99 degrees once, when I had H1N1 flu.

I dug the thermometer out of the clutter at the bottom of the bathroom vanity drawer and popped it in my mouth. A minute later, it buzzed. When I took it out, I was surprised to see the electronic digits read 101.8. Huh. I guess this might be my problem. So I once again retrieved the number for Dr. Smith's answering service, reluctant to call after office hours, but alarmed by the numbers on the thermometer, and described my symptoms to the receptionist.

Dr. Smith called me back a few minutes later.

How's the surgical area look? he asked after I repeated my symptoms.

Well, I said, pretty red.

Does it look redder than it did a few days ago when I saw you in the office?

Well. Yes, probably. Actually, now that you mention it, it's bright red. And a bit streaky. And yes, it's painful. But it's been pretty red and painful all along, I added hopefully.

I think you may be getting an infection, he said. I'm going to call in two antibiotic prescriptions for you that you should begin tonight, and I want to see you at eight a.m. tomorrow morning.

Jeff, ever at the ready, went out to Walgreens to get the prescriptions, and I hunkered down on the sofa to watch Star Trek reruns with Elena. When I went to bed that night, I lay awake wondering if pulling the drains too early had anything to do with my newest plight. There was, of course, no way to know. And it was too late to know it anyway.

•   •   •   •   •

Thus began the four-month period I will call The Troubles. Also known as One Damn Thing After Another. Also known as the anti-medical establishment conditioning program, because by the end, I never wanted to step foot in another clinic or hospital again.

Had I understood in August 2010, when I chose so cavalierly to begin breast reconstruction, the possible consequences of that choice, I would have paused a bit longer to consider. Was I willing to sacrifice hundreds of hours from my remaining life, be it one year or fifty, to the enterprise of having fake breasts? Was that sacrifice of time, not to mention the financial and other resources I consumed, an acceptable price for the ability to walk around the occasional locker room naked without feeling self-conscious? With the time I ultimately devoted to the reconstruction process and resulting medical care, including the alien eye disaster of the previous winter, I could maybe have built a rocket to Saturn. Or orchestrated world peace. Or at least have written a bestselling novel. That's how it feels, anyway.

But, although in our heads, we may finagle the events in our lives into patterns that will help us predict what happens next, we can't know the future. And even though the fine print on the consent forms warns us about all the possible catastrophic consequences of our choices, we don't believe they will happen to us. If we've done nothing to deserve a bad outcome, if we've lived a good life, been compliant, paid the bills on time, we can expect good results. Right? Bad things only happen to bad people. Right?

Early the next morning, Jeff drove me back up to Dr. Smith's office in the suburbs, where Ashley immediately ushered us into an exam room. The office was peaceful and empty at eight a.m., a contrast to the usual commotion of patients coming and going for appointments every ten minutes, and I felt a vague shame at calling attention to myself outside of business hours. My temperature was down, maybe because of the Tylenol I'd been popping every four hours since the previous night, but the streaky redness seemed to be getting worse. I also had fairly frequent waves of dizziness and weakness that made me need to sit, lest I fall.

After taking a look, and extracting some cloudy, dark fluid from the site with a syringe, Dr. Smith explained that he thought I might be developing an infection, but since we'd caught it early, we could *probably* still save the reconstruction. If we waited and a more serious infection developed, it could mean losing the migrated tissue and the implant from the surgery and possibly risk a more dangerous systemic infection, which can be life-threatening. Before I really had time to digest this, Ashley was on the phone with the hospital to see what floor I should report to for my room assignment, Dr. Smith was phoning in treatment orders, and Jeff and I were packing up our belongings and getting ready to move the car over to the hospital parking ramp.

Well. How did I get here?

A sense of unreality set in. It's odd, walking to the fourth-floor ward of a suburban hospital at 8:30 a.m. and being shown to your room, as if you've crossed an ocean and multiple time zones and are checking in early to an exotic hotel so you can grab a nap before sight-seeing. Then stripping off your street clothes and stuffing them in a closet, so you can don the blue and white, over-washed hospital gown, whose inadequacy for covering your ass is so prosaic it's not even worth mentioning. Then pulling on the creepy, rubber-soled hospital socks, because it's summer and you wore sandals and the nurses insist on footgear. Then climbing between the stiff white hospital sheets in the middle of the morning, and settling in to see what happens next. I was glad I'd brought my book.

•   •   •   •   •

And so began five days of hospital hijinks.

Soon my room filled up with a parade of people wanting to poke me and prod me and have me pull open my inadequate gown so they could view my ever-reddening chest. A lab tech drew blood for the multi-day culture that would reveal what particular bacteria had taken up residence in my surgical site. I peed into a cup and handed it over for testing. An infectious disease doctor came by to have a look and get acquainted since we were clearly going to spend some time together in the next few weeks. An IV was started, so I could get antibiotics delivered straight into my bloodstream.

I came to understand that I would be staying there, hooked up to an IV delivering a variety of antibiotics, until the blood culture results came back and they knew exactly what to treat me with. That could take several days.

I'm allergic to sulfa drugs (internal and external hives; trouble breathing) and drugs in the penicillin family (minor hives, but risky), so the antibiotic choices were limited. And when they started pumping Cipro, a third powerful antibiotic option, through my IV line that morning, the veins in my left hand lit up bright red, like the electrified circulatory system in the mannequin at the science museum. So out came the Cipro, and, adding a little extra kick, the IV had to be moved to the right side, just to be safe.

Sometime in the afternoon, I settled into a diet of IV Vancomycin, oral Cipro, and bad hospital food. The pizza I'd ordered for lunch arrived burnt beyond edibility. The salad consisted of iceberg lettuce with a shaving of limp carrot, leaving me to despair over the fresh, crunchy organic greens tucked away in my fridge at home. Even the cookie was hard and tasteless. The IV pump seemed to beep uncontrollably every fifteen minutes, and the staff's response rate was glacial.

Jeff had departed in the morning to tend to work responsibilities, and he would return later, bringing something edible for dinner. But my optimistic mood from a few days earlier soon deteriorated into a bleak realization that I could be here for a week. I began to think I could quite possibly either starve to death or die of boredom.

When Dr. Smith came by to check on me at the end of the day, he told me it was possible he would want to go in surgically, remove the expander, and replace it with a shiny new, uninfected one. But he'd keep me posted. He left, and Jeff and Elena arrived with dinner but didn't stay too long. And soon I was once again alone with my IV and my iPod, dialing the playlist back to *Adagio for Strings*.

• • • • •

I awoke at about 6 a.m. on Saturday, when an orderly arrived to take me to surgery.

What surgery? I asked.

You're going into surgery at seven a.m., he said.

No, I said. My doctor said we'd *talk* about surgery. We haven't talked about it yet. I'm not ready to go into surgery.

Well, we'll just take you down there, he said. You can talk to him down there.

I hesitated. But what was I going to do? Cross my arms and pout? Refuse to get in the chair? I wished fervently for Jeff to appear and be the voice of reason, to ask all the right questions and help me with the answers. But I knew it was too early for him to show up.

So I got in the chair, and the orderly wheeled me downstairs to the same day-surgery unit where I'd had my alien-eye surgery in February. In the surgery unit, a flurry of activity ensued. An anesthesiologist came and went, my IV was checked, nurses came to take my vitals and tuck in blankets. Before I knew it, I'd been prepped to go into the surgery suite.

I lay stoic and defeated in my cubicle. The warm blankets didn't calm my jitters, and the bright lights hurt my eyes. I didn't know if this was the right thing to do, but I didn't have what it would take to fight it. I hadn't been able to grab my phone before the orderly whisked me out of my room, so I couldn't call Jeff to let him know this was happening.

Finally, Dr. Smith appeared. He explained that he had considered my situation and done some research, and he'd decided he needed to go ahead and replace the expander and hope for the best. In his usual careful way, he described the risks and benefits of the surgery, then patted my foot and said he'd see me in the OR.

It wasn't that I disagreed. I trusted his judgment. But I hadn't had time to consider this decision, and I had no one with whom I could talk it through. And frankly, I'd become increasingly nervous about the procedures at this particular hospital. Shouldn't someone have told me last night that this was scheduled, so I would have had time to wrap my head around it? Had rogue operating room bacteria during the original surgery caused this infection, and should I be worried about that? Why had Jeff been able to tap idly on a mobile computer station left in my hospital room and see other patients' records spring to life? And how can you cook a frozen pizza (perilously close to inedible by its very nature), which requires no cooking skill whatsoever, so badly as to make it completely inedible? And why would you think it was okay to serve it to anyone once you had? If the same level of care applied in the OR as in the kitchen, I was in trouble.

But who's going to argue with the surgeon, especially when the orderlies are tapping their toes, impatient to wheel you in? So they wheeled me through the familiar double doors, the rumble of the gurney echoing off the sterile walls. And I counted backward from one hundred into oblivion.

When I woke up, I was crying. I don't know when I'd started crying, having been anesthetized and all, but tears were running down my face, and I was alone in the recovery area. I couldn't believe this was happening. That this ordeal, which had promised to come full-circle within a pleasingly precise calendar year, July to July, had veered into territory I never expected. I didn't want breasts this badly. I could have managed without them. My well-meaning, if misguided friend had been right: I was pretty much finished with them. I'd thought it was going to be easy, a road to wholeness that would help me spin past cancer and move on with my life. But here we were, several unanticipated surgeries later, not to mention the multiple minor cut and stitch sessions, and there was not an end in sight.

Eventually, a nurse appeared to check on me. But apparently, they schedule all the harried, insensitive nurses in the day-surgery area on Saturdays, because this one, like the post-surgery nurse in February, was in a hurry to move me out. Not unlike the radiation tech a few months earlier, she noticed me crying as she checked my vitals, and said: You're fine. There's nothing to cry about. Then she logged my stats on the computer and walked away.

So many uses of the word "fine." Sometimes so right, sometimes so very wrong. During that cancer year, I told myself and everyone around me that I was fine at least a thousand times. And I'd been telling the truth. From day to day, even during this difficult time in my life, even coping with cancer and unexpected surgeries and disappointment and despair, I was, mostly, fine.

And I now know that Dr. McCarthy was right when she told me I was going to be fine. In the big picture, whether I live another year or another fifty years, I know I will be fine. I've lived a full life. I have continued to be grateful for each additional day. I consider every year I've lived since my diagnosis to be a gift.

But that moment in the recovery room was one of the few moments in the cancerland jungle when I was *not* fine. I needed someone to hold my hand and tell me the struggle was worth it. That there would still be dog walks and state parks and dinner parties and music and sweet corn and high-end bakeries, once I got through this part. That my kids and my spouse and my family and friends all wanted me around, for a long, long time, and I just needed to get through one more thing, eyes on the road ahead.

But that nurse didn't know that when she told me I was fine. And when I asked her to check on whether my husband was there and could come sit with me, she told me he would meet me back in my room. I didn't know if that meant he was there, but I couldn't see him. Or he wasn't at the hospital yet. Or he was fed up with the whole cancer thing and was on his way to Brazil with the cute divorcee. I wouldn't blame him. But the nurse didn't seem willing to figure it out for me. So I lay in my recovery cubicle and cried.

Eventually, an orderly wheeled me up to my room, me crying the whole way. Back in bed, I pulled the stiff hospital sheets over my head, shut my eyes, and drifted off.

When I woke up, Jeff was sitting in the chair by my bed, computer on his lap. He'd brought pastries from my favorite French bakery, and the grease-stained bag crackled familiarly as he drew out an almond croissant and set it on a napkin on my tray table. I pulled myself up and reached for the croissant. As I ate, a shower of golden pastry flakes rained down, embellishing my faded blue and white gown and the snowy sheets below. Between bites, I looked at Jeff and tried to smile.

•   •   •   •   •

Saturday passed quietly after that. Mostly, the nurses left me alone because there was not much to be done, I suppose. When a private room became available, I moved. So moving broke up the afternoon. I could now watch bad TV without disturbing a roommate and talk freely on my new iPhone to friends and relatives who'd heard of my plight and were texting or calling to check in. Mostly I slept or listened to music or played solitaire on my computer.

Sunday morning, Jeff arrived with more croissants and an update on his Saturday evening with Elena. He settled in next to me for the day, as I checked email and fielded the morning round of nurses and aides.

Around 8 a.m., Dr. Smith appeared. We put away the computers and the pastries so we could take in the report about Saturday's surgery. Jeff adjusted his chair, which screeched slightly on the tile floor, to better view Dr. Smith. I brushed the crumbs off my gown.

I removed the infected expander, Dr. Smith said. It was starting to show signs of the bacterial "slime" that begins to form around an infected area. Then I flushed the area with ten gallons of saline to wash out the site.

As he described the surgery, I could feel the bacterial slime on my fingers, like the film on the bottom of the dog's water bowl when I haven't cleaned it properly for a few days. I imagined ten gallons of bacterial tea, *my* bacterial tea, flooding the OR, swirling down a drain in the surgery suite floor and making its way to the Mississippi. I'm sure it's not like that, I thought. But I wondered where it ends up.

I had to install a new expander, to restore the sterile area, Dr. Smith explained. But overall, the surgery went really well. You can probably go home on Tuesday, after the bacterial culture is back. Then we'll know for sure you're on the right antibiotic. Until then, we'll keep you on the IV Vancomycin that you've been on since Friday morning, which should treat the infection.

I looked at Jeff, who looked at the IV pole, which had been standing, abandoned, in the corner of the room since yesterday morning. I looked back at Dr. Smith.

But I haven't been receiving any drugs since the surgery, I said. They unhooked the IV line when they brought me back up here yesterday, and I haven't been hooked up again since.

For once, Dr. Smith's usual professional demeanor showed a slight crack. I thought I saw alarm—or was it just surprise?—in his eyes. He glanced at the IV pole in the corner, then down at my hand, where the IV needle was secured with tape, but the set-up was unencumbered by the usual octopus of tubes.

You haven't received any antibiotics since yesterday morning?

Nope, I said. Just my Tamoxifen and standard sleeping aids, by mouth last night.

Jeff nodded his agreement.

Pause.

I'll be back, Dr. Smith said. He turned and left the room.

Jeff and I looked at each other.

Soon the room was a-flurry with people drawing more blood, hanging IV bags, and connecting me back to the octopus of tubes. In between visits, Jeff would say, Huh. This is interesting. Then he'd return to tapping away on his computer.

Dr. Smith spent the rest of his Sunday getting to the bottom of why a patient hospitalized for an infection had, for over twenty-four hours, not received the antibiotics her doctor had ordered as treatment. Of course, none of this was my fault, other than in a broadly existential way. But to this day, I feel the need to apologize to his family. I don't think that's how he planned to spend his Sunday. I think he planned to toss the ball around in the yard with his kids, maybe go on a bike ride to the lake. I imagined him, instead, pacing through the hospital in his scrubs thinking, Shit! Why does this kind of thing always happen with lawyers?

Despite my conversations with the patient care representative, the infectious disease doctor, Dr. Smith, and various other people who came through my room in the next few days, I never did get the full story of what happened. Something about the medication order being canceled in the pharmacy, so it didn't get sent up, and the nurses didn't notice...or whatever. I certainly hadn't noticed. But then I was post-anesthesia and not a medical professional. It wasn't my job to notice.

Sunday afternoon, Jeff spent some time arguing with the on-call infectious disease doctor, who was not nearly as pleasant and reasonable as *my* infectious disease doctor, who'd been assigned to me on Friday. *My* infectious disease doctor grew up in Northfield, two blocks from our house, in a lovely brick bungalow I walked past every morning with Ruby, and went to Carleton, where Jeff taught and Sam went to school, so was obviously a superior person. This on-call doctor insisted that somehow the antibiotic lapse wasn't a problem, which Jeff was having none of.

As they argued, I looked on from my bed, so grateful today to have an advocate, someone who was willing to take on a contentious doctor *and* show up at the hospital with my favorite baked goods several days in a row. Could I ask for a better life partner? I settled back with a sigh.

Possibly, technically, the doctor may have been right. Maybe the missing day of antibiotics was not a big deal. I did get better, after all, and he's the infection expert.

But a word to the wise doctor: at a minimum, it *looks* really bad to mess up by failing to give antibiotics to a patient hospitalized with a potentially dangerous infection. I'd say arguing about it is not the best choice. I'd say the better choice is to tell the patient: I'm sorry this happened, but I'm confident you will be okay. I'd say this might just help the patient feel better, or even *get* better.

They should teach you that in medical school.

Despite all this, I felt good on Sunday, antibiotics pumping once again into my arm. I perked up when I realized that three days confined to a hospital bed presented an opportunity to organize my classical music files in iTunes, a time-consuming job I'd neglected for over a year. My spirits were also lifted by visits from friends anxious to cheer me up. Jeff's parents came for a while, Carolyn stopped in for a lovely, lazy Sunday afternoon chat, and Jackie, who has no patience with bad food, brought a variety of delicious organic salads, enough to feed me for several days.

There's been no naturally occurring Stupid Metaphor for a while, so here's a made up one. I rode out the tsunami of tears, which had threatened to drown me on Saturday, on Sunday's surfboard of generosity and friendship, which kept me floating toward shore. But I mean it.

•   •   •   •   •

The lab results, which came back on Tuesday morning, showed that I had a standard hospital staph infection, treatable with IV Vancomycin, the drug I'd been receiving (mostly!) since Friday. I did not delve into the biology, but apparently standard oral antibiotic therapy would not combat this kind of systemic infection. So Tuesday around noon, a portable IV-insertion specialist showed up in my room to install an IV line into the soft inner cave of my left upper arm, through which I would administer my own drugs for the next month. A home health nurse would come to our house later that day to bring the necessary supplies, review the protocol with me, and help me run the first batch. She would then check up on me every few days at home.

We packed up, and it was not unlike leaving the hotel room in the alternate time zone. Making sure we had the computers and small devices and all their cords and accessories. Retrieving the dirty clothing from the back of the closet and stuffing it in the suitcase. Checking the back of the bathroom door one more time for a stray t-shirt or bathrobe. I refused the wheelchair because I felt perfectly fine, and we walked to the elevator and out to the parking garage.

The home health nurse arrived later in the afternoon as promised, bearing a load of equipment. Tubes and lines in sterile packets. Alcohol wipes, rolls of gauze, and stretchy armbands to cover the IV site and keep the tubes in place. A large Styrofoam cooler filled with pre-bagged antibiotics. The supplies took over the kitchen island, spilled onto the dining room table, filled the refrigerator drawer usually reserved for vegetables. The cats, undisciplined about kitchen counter etiquette, jumped up and sniffed the plastic bags and batted at the enticingly snaky tube as the nurse removed it from its packaging. She shooed them away, pursed her mouth, sniffed, and brushed the fur bunnies off the island with a firm hand.

The nurse instructed me to administer one full bag of medicine twice a day. Each treatment would take a couple of hours. While the bag of medicine fed through the line and into my arm, I could wear a fanny pack, always my favorite fashion accessory, to carry the bag around. Don't crimp the line, and be sure to run all the medicine out every time. Yes, ma'am.

The visit was unsettling. For the first time in all of this, I felt the humid, sticky breath of old age and dependency on my neck. I was a ward of the health system, not competent to monitor my own treatment. I might as well crawl into bed and call it a life.

Administering the medicine twice a day proved to be inconvenient, but workable. I went back to work on Wednesday, the day after I arrived home, eager to prep for the upcoming semester. I got my teaching materials ready and worked on a conference presentation, scheduled for September. I chose the topics for my magazine column and worked on an article with a colleague, which we'd started the summer before, but had been preempted by cancer. I looked forward to the upcoming school year and the promise the new semester always holds.

The following Monday morning, a week after my hospital release, the home health nurse came to the house at 8 a.m. to check me over and make sure I was in compliance. I was anxious to get out the door because I had a meeting at work around ten o'clock, to work on the cancer-delayed article, and I didn't want to be late. My lunch was packed, and my commuting tea was brewing in its travel mug on the kitchen island.

The nurse instructed me to sit on a stool at the island, then methodically examined my IV site, changed the line, and inventoried my supplies. While she worked on my left arm, I used my right hand to check email on my phone.

After she changed the line, she poked and prodded my left arm a bit. I think your forearm looks a little puffy. See that swelling there?

No, I don't think so, I replied, looking up from my phone. I don't see any swelling.

Hmm. I think maybe there's a little swelling, she said, working my fingers back and forth.

No, I'm quite sure there's no swelling, I said. I really need to go to work now.

I tried to pull my arm away from her, but she held on, turning it back and forth.

Well, she said, finally letting go. I think there's some swelling. I'm going to go back to the office and talk to my supervisor and see what she thinks. I'll be in touch.

She packed up her equipment, and I herded her out the door. Then I grabbed my bags, enticed the dog outside with a bone-shaped biscuit, and jumped in my car to head out the corn corridor to the highway. About twenty minutes up the highway, my phone rang, interrupting the music that had been playing through my kick-ass sound system.

It was, of course, the nurse.

Mary, she said. Where are you? You need to go to the nearest hospital emergency room and be evaluated for a blood clot.

I told her I was about ten miles south of Burnsville, near the hospital where I'd had my radiation treatments in the spring. Then I argued. I really needed to go to work, I said. Could I go to the ER in Saint Paul, after my morning meeting? Could I go later, when I got back to Northfield?

But she was adamant that I could be in a dangerous situation.

Sufficiently freaked out, I pulled onto the Burnsville exit ramp, took the familiar right onto Nicollet Avenue, and headed towards the neon red Emergency sign, swearing all the way. On my way through the parking lot, I left a message for my colleague saying I wouldn't make the ten o'clock meeting and wondering if the article was doomed to incomplete article purgatory, a hazard of academic life.

At the ER desk, I explained my situation to the intake nurse, who immediately ushered me back to a cubicle and had me strip from the waist up. Familiarity with this ritual had definitely bred contempt, not comfort. At least the blue hospital gowns were adequate here.

Then I was stranded. I had not expected any leisure time that day, so I had not brought a book. There were no magazines in the cubicle. I was deep in the bowels of the hospital, so I had no phone reception, and could not even get a text out to tell Jeff where I was and what was happening. My only occupation choices were the horrors of daytime TV, Dora the Explorer videos, or Boggle on my phone. I'd left my lunch in the car.

After some hapless waiting and half-hearted Boggle games, followed by ultrasound imaging, it turned out I had a blood clot near my left clavicle. Blood clots are dangerous. They can break loose, travel through your arteries to your lungs, lodge themselves in the mysterious recesses of your alveoli, and kill you. The clot appeared to have been caused by the IV line, so there was agreement all around that the line had to come out. Tamoxifen, cancer, and a history of chemotherapy can also make you susceptible to blood clots. Apparently, my general good health, low cholesterol, low blood pressure, and habitual compliance, were no match for this axis of evil. So here I was.

Nothing like the threat of sudden death by pulmonary embolism to take your mind off cancer.

It took several hours for the ER doctor to contact Dr. Smith, who was in surgery, and for Dr. Smith to contact my infectious disease doctor, who was on hospital rounds, and for all three doctors to confer and decide what to do with me. In the meantime, I felt like I'd been disappeared into a North Korean prison, where my family would never find me. My phone battery was approaching critical levels from all the Boggle games, lunchtime had long passed with only apple juice and graham crackers on offer, and my spirits were pretty low.

Around two o'clock, the doctors weighed in. The solution was actually quite simple. Take out the IV line and put me on oral antibiotics and a blood thinner to clear the blood clot.

Oral antibiotics?! If an oral antibiotic existed that would treat my infection and not cause me to swell up with hives, why had I been messing around with this IV line for the past week?

At this point, we entered into a world of antibiotic politics and science that I do not fully understand. But I'm willing to trust that the medical professionals in charge of antibiotic policy at the Centers for Disease Control know what they're doing. Apparently, a few antibiotics exist that can only be prescribed by infectious disease specialists, in hospitals, to combat MRSA-type creatures that will otherwise take over the earth and bring an end to humanity as we know it. These antibiotics are tightly controlled, so they remain armed and ready to defeat our microscopic enemies. But because I was at the end of the antibiotic line, with no other options, my infectious disease doctor could prescribe one of them for me. And so a magic pill called Zyvox entered my life.

I was so relieved. Lucky me, to have a blood clot. My life would be so much easier with the nice white oval pills rather than the IV line and the fanny pack. True, I had to inject myself in the belly with blood thinners twice a day over the next several weeks, while gradually switching over to an oral medication that would do the job instead. But that seemed preferable to the IV line and tackle that had encumbered me for over a week. So I left the hospital late that afternoon, humming, and headed back down the highway, preparing to tell the latest harrowing tale to my family.

Chapter Twenty

Just as it's impossible to know what caused my cancer, it's impossible to know what caused The Troubles that began when I started taking Zyvox. Given everything that had happened to me since the July surgery, I was now on medical appointment rounds that included regular visits with the plastic surgeon (for the Growing-up Skipper treatment), the oncologist (to monitor the blood clot), and the infectious disease doctor (to make sure I wasn't dead yet). Also, blood had to be drawn at the hospital lab every few days for four to six weeks to measure the blood thinners in my system. I was also seeing the physical therapist three times a week to regain function on my right side, post-surgery.

In the next few weeks, my body began to protest in ways I could not have predicted, sending me into a stupefying treatment whirlwind. First, I contracted a urinary tract infection that would seem to clear up with a course of antibiotics, only to come raging back a few days later. This went on week after week, for several months, requiring doctor visits with whoever was on routine infection duty at the clinic and round after round of various antibiotics.

Meanwhile, my joints swelled and ached, making getting out of bed in the morning painful. Maybe a lingering side effect of chemo. Maybe a new a side effect of the various antibiotics. My perineum began to peel and bleed (forget you read that if you're squeamish about lady parts), making daily life uncomfortable and the prospect of a sex life challenging, and necessitating a round of visits with the gynecologist. Maybe the Tamoxifen, maybe the antibiotics. My jawbone began to necrotize, sending bone shards through my gums to slice the tender underside of my tongue. My dentist had recently retired, so I consulted his newly hired replacement, who was twelve years old and had been in practice for ten minutes, who sent me immediately to an oral surgeon, who didn't quite know what to make of it, but told me to come back in two weeks. The breast infection looked like maybe it was recurring, so I took a second round of Zyvox, afraid of what would happen if I didn't.

Not having enough to do, or thinking that one more appointment wouldn't matter, I made an appointment for an eye exam, which I'd neglected for several years. The exam revealed that I had a bleed in the back of my eye, possibly a result of the blood thinners. Come back in two weeks for a recheck, my optometrist told me.

Over the fall, I had at least three medical visits a week for four months. My dance card was completely full. I kept the local medical community profitable single-handedly. And by the time December rolled around, I was sick of it.

In some ways, this parade of endless, inexplicable maladies made me more miserable than the previous fall's mastectomy surgery and chemotherapy. There didn't seem to be an explanation or a way to make it stop. And people don't bring casseroles and prayer shawls because your bladder is on fire, your lady parts are inexplicably ulcerating, and you can't bend your toes. Nor did I really want to talk about how miserable I was. So I couldn't catch the wave of sympathy that came with the initial cancer diagnosis, or even the surgeries that followed. I couldn't plausibly stay home from work, because resting up just didn't help much, and, besides, I didn't want to explain, even to my closest friends. At least working got my mind off my troubles.

I think many of us find ourselves in this same space when we encounter tough spots in our lives, regular old tough spots that don't involve cancer. We may have a particularly heavy inventory of mundane ills—maybe neck pain *and* sciatica *and* gloomy adolescent children *and* a partner who doesn't know how to connect *and* aging parents—and from day to day, it's really hard, and we're miserable. Maybe even more miserable than our neighbor with cancer, who is, deservedly, getting all the attention. But because cancer—The Big C— has this special place in our pantheon of Troubles, when it gets named, the spotlight shifts to the afflicted, and the support system rallies. In fact, many people with these invisible daily ills could also benefit from casseroles and prayer shawls and daily check-ins, maybe even more so. We all have troubles during our lives that fall somewhere on the sliding scale towards cancer. But we don't have a way to label our Troubles in public or to ask for what we need. Or we think we're weak because we need anything at all. So we suffer alone, in silence, and wait for it to get better.

Maybe cancer has a special place in our catalogue of suffering because when you have it, you may in fact die. And when you're in the position of possibly dying, people naturally and generously want to reach out to you and care for you. We all circle around death, averting our eyes, yet pulled by its inexorable gravity. But, despite my anxiety about dying, and despite my particularly virulent case of cancer, I was still statistically more likely to die of commuting than of cancer. And potential death by commuting does not garner much attention from your support community. I suppose because you have a choice about risking death by commuting, but you have little choice about death by cancer.

Right?

It's a puzzle.

In any case, none of my doctors wanted to venture a guess about why this cascade of symptoms happened to me that fall. As I view it now, it all began with the Zyvox. But I was assured that these were not possible side effects of that drug. I considered going off the Tamoxifen to see if my symptoms improved, but that just put me at greater risk for more cancer. And, in the past year, I'd been on such a potent cocktail of chemotherapy, antibiotics, anti-nausea drugs, anti-estrogen drugs, immune system support drugs, and blood thinners, all stirred together with a good heaping of stress and alternative medicine supplements, that it truly was impossible to connect any one symptom with any one cause. I think my body just couldn't cope with the overload anymore and was finally speaking up: Enough. Stop. Please.

So I did, mostly. My next surgery, to remove the expanders on both sides and replace them with permanent implants, was scheduled for early December 2011. I needed to be off the blood thinners for a week before surgery, and I told my oncologist that I did not plan to resume taking them, against her recommendation. I stopped the Tamoxifen, damn the consequences. I finished up all the UTI antibiotics and drank gallons of water, determined to avoid another round. I stopped all supplements and decided to forgo even Tylenol and ibuprofen for a while. I did a lot of yoga, canceled all doctor appointments except those required for the upcoming surgery, and did everything I could to reduce my stress and find some peace.

•　　•　　•　　•　　•

Sometimes, when you're looking for peace, you find it in places you don't expect. I found peace in Methodist Hospital, at the Mayo Clinic, because Sam was in crisis and needed to have his colon removed. And when your child is so heartbreakingly ill and thin that you can hardly look at him without tearing up, everything else in your life disappears, even cancer and the specter of pulmonary embolism.

Sam came home at Thanksgiving that year in bad shape. He'd been a Crohn's Disease trooper for over six years, ever good-natured about spending half his life in the bathroom. But the ordeal had taken its toll on him, and he was sick and discouraged. He had reached the end of the road on treatment options, and this horrendous disease severely limited his life. His doctor told him clearly: you are the sickest person I will see today, and I see a lot of sick people. You need to have this surgery.

So in early December 2011, within ten days, I had surgery to install my permanent implants, Elena had her wisdom teeth extracted, a previously scheduled, now inconvenient, event, and Sam made the decision to have his colon surgically removed.

My surgery was an outpatient, one-day affair, a week after Thanksgiving, in a surprisingly light and airy, fifth-floor surgery suite, with windows that looked out on the school playground across the street. A surgery suite with windows, not in the bowels of the hospital! This was more healing than aromatherapy and hand massage put together. I recovered over the weekend, back to full service by Monday, so I could take Elena to her date with the oral surgeon. The free pint of ice cream they handed her on the way out did little to compensate her for her woes.

Our sofas were full. In fact, we were one short. Sam huddled under the pink kitty blanket on the green sofa, rising only to make his way to the bathroom, Elena huddled under her blue stars and moons comforter on the brown sofa, unable to talk or eat, and I slotted myself in where I could by someone's feet. Jeff sat in his chair and wielded the remote, Ruby panting at his side, waiting patiently for someone to muster the energy for a walk. In the afternoons, I left them to their dumb TV and napped upstairs, conserving my energy so I could later make strawberry smoothies for Elena and Campbell's chicken noodle soup for Sam.

Let me just say: poor Elena. Not only had much of her teenage life been eclipsed by her brother's illness, and her senior year in high school overshadowed by her mother's cancer, now we could hardly muster the attention to fetch sherbet and ice packs, and watch dumb TV with her while she recovered from this painful rite of passage. She had started college that fall, and despite my Troubles, we'd shown up for move-in day and Parent's Weekend and the other rituals of freshman year. We did our best, but it couldn't be enough. And here, on her first break home from her new adventure, it was worse than ever. She's a strong person, and I know she'll recover from all this neglect by the time she's fifty. But in the meantime, I felt like I owed her several trips to London and Paris and anywhere else she wanted to go.

A few days later, after several days of familial couch occupation, when Sam's crisis came to a head, Jeff and I began trading off trips to the Mayo Clinic, in Rochester, Minnesota, where Sam was receiving treatment and would have his surgery.

The hour drive to Rochester is beautiful when the cornfields are blanketed in snow and the sun rides low and golden in the sky. The crows, immune to the cold, gather in trees along the rolling hills, keeping watch over the tidy farms tucked in for the winter. A few late migrating geese honk overhead, hurrying to catch the jet stream heading south. We'd made this drive in all seasons taking Sam to appointments, sometimes daily when he was hospitalized. That December, I spent many hours speeding down the highway, Sam dozing in the seat beside me, thinking about how much I was ready to move on. Ready to move on from cancer. Ready to help Sam move on from this crisis that no young adult should have to endure.

I pulled the straw to accompany Sam the day of his surgery. Jeff would stay home with Elena, then we would switch late in the day. The procedure was scheduled early, so we headed down the highway in the dark, the stars charting our way from above.

We went through the now so familiar surgery prep hoops—trading civilian clothes for the blue and white hospital gown, tolerating the invasion of an IV insertion, answering the anesthesiologist's questions, checking in with the surgeon to make sure we knew what was up. This time, I was the one in the nearby chair, holding my tears at bay. I did what I could to keep Sam's spirits up. I took a picture of him and sent it to Jeff—the last we would have of him with his body intact. In the picture, he is vampire-pale, and his cheekbones would make a Calvin Klein model proud. He huddles under his own mountain of warm blankets, and I can see the worry in his eyes, the same worry I'm sure Jeff had seen in my eyes eighteen months before. But Sam didn't cry.

They wheeled Sam through his own double doors, and for a minute, I envied him the oblivion that would bring. The pain of watching my child suffer was far worse than anything I had experienced in the last two years. I would have done anything to take this away from him.

I left the hospital and went to explore downtown Rochester for a couple of hours, because what else could I do? I was done with sad, sad waiting rooms full of sad, sad people, even when I was on the non-patient side. Downtown, I bought some clothes, signifying, a la my friend Angie, my intent to live a long time in my new body. I tried on shoes and looked at the high-end art galleries that court Mayo's more exclusive clientele. As I sat in the dim, underground shopping maze that connects the clinic with the commercial district, eating my frozen yogurt and worrying about Sam, the surgeon called to say he was done and all was well. I dumped the frozen yogurt in the trash and hurried back to the hospital.

I waited for Sam to come up from recovery in a beautiful, state-of-the-art private hospital room in a wing that had been open only a few weeks. It was clean, shiny, and flashy with gadgets, but also comfortingly under-lit and quiet. Many of the rooms were empty in this week before Christmas. The nurses were freshly hired for this new wing, corn-fed recent graduates from nearby nursing programs, mostly in their early- to mid-twenties. They were competent, energetic, and fresh-faced. What could better fuel the recovery of an adorable twenty-one-year-old guy than his own stock of private nurses, eager to bring him sherbet and chat about his internet feed?

The orderlies wheeled Sam in, and the state-of-the-art equipment kicked in. No "one, two three, lift" in this room. Instead, a clever robotic contraption installed in the ceiling hooked to the sling-like surface of the gurney and lifted him ever so gently into the bed. Sam looked about as big around as my arm, a mere sapling when he should have been a strong young oak by now. As I stroked his hair and cried, he came around a bit and assured me he was fine. I cried some more as he slept, grateful that perhaps his ordeal was over, hopeful that he could once again live a normal life in which he felt good, could swing dance to his heart's content, spend hours on a movie set without a bathroom, and go on dates unimpeded.

We inhabited that peaceful room together for many hours over the next week, sharing that space of healing, interrupted only by one of the fresh-faced nurses needing to check vitals or help Sam out of bed for a short walk. I read a book, or just looked out the window, replaying in my head the ordeal of the past eighteen months. Sam slept or read on his computer or watched movies, insulated with headphones. Occasionally, small troupes of his friends showed up, just as my friends had shown up for me. I would leave the room to go sit in the nearby family lounge, enjoying their voices and laughter from down the hall, knowing Sam would have what he needed as he moved into his adult life. Every 24 hours or so Jeff would arrive, and after an hour together in the room, we would pass the parental baton so I could go home, take a shower, and hang out with Elena.

As I sat in that quiet room with Sam and looked out at the darkened streets of Rochester, where a few holidays lights twinkled in the night, I realized I had never thought Crohn's Disease was in any way something he had brought on himself, or deserved, or could control. When Crohn's Disease pounced from the thicket and ambushed him, he was an innocent —only fourteen years old, and not a culpable bone in his body. He'd done nothing to strike out, unless I believed that an excess of video games and a few toddler tantrums counted, which I did not. Why did these ideas that *I* was responsible for my cancer, or that *I* somehow had control over my illness, continue to lurk in the damp caverns of my brain, when I so clearly did not believe the same about Sam?

Maybe it was time to give up those ideas, which seemed rooted in a youthful aversion to uncertainty, a desire for a magical world that would ease my way if only I knew the right spells. I'd felt uncertain about my own ability to cope with life's crises, and certain that, left to flail on my own, I would make a mistake. If I could accept that I am enough, that I can trust myself to cope, no matter what comes my way, then I could truly embrace the life in front of me, confident that freedom to choose my course would serve me well.

I saw that I had done the best I could—with Sam's illness, my own illness, the complications for my family—just as Sam had done the best he could. And now I envisioned Sam gaining strength as his body learned to handle food again, allowing him to reclaim his life. I envisioned Elena moving forward in her new life at college, blossoming into the confident young woman we knew she could be. I envisioned

Jeff and me together making a post-cancer, post-children-at-home life exploring new pleasures and expanded opportunities. I would make mistakes along the way. But the possibilities beckoned.

It felt like an opportunity to begin anew. The new year, 2012—a pleasingly round, balanced number, suggesting happy possibility, a relief after the disquieting prime number year of 2011—was about to begin. After surgery, Sam would no longer need monthly infusions or daily medications, or any intervention at all, once he learned to manage his colostomy. He could essentially be done with doctors for a while. And, my permanent implants now in place, I could do the same. I could choose, or not, to proceed with the final reconstruction touches, the cosmetic flourishes that many women, finished with needles and surgeons, forgo. We could start the year fresh, putting the frenzy of medical intervention behind us, ready to begin the next phase of our lives.

I sat in the silence and opened my heart to whatever happened next, with gratitude, an open mind, and no expectations. Because here, home in this life, with all of its troubles and gifts, was where I wanted to be.

Chapter Twenty-One

Although I found some peace in that hospital room with Sam, I wasn't quite done with cancer. After a six-month hiatus from doctors and hospitals and medical interventions, I decided to finish the reconstruction job with Dr. Smith. I made an appointment for nipple reconstruction surgery, the penultimate piece of the reconstruction puzzle. A few months after that, I could have the final touch—the whipped cream and cherry on the sundae: tattooed areolas.

Many women forgo this whole reconstruction endgame, content just to avoid bra inserts for the rest of their lives, not concerned about the prospect of blankly staring boobs when naked in the locker room. I just wanted to complete the circle and feel like I'd made it to the finish line. Cancer had not made me less goal-oriented.

Nipple reconstruction involves cutting a flap in the existing skin, stitching it up into a raised cylinder far larger than a natural nipple, and then waiting for it to shrink down into a perfectly round button scar. So I returned to the windowed fifth-floor surgery suite for nipple reconstruction surgery. This was a causal day-surgery center, and Dr. Smith worked on my chest with no draping or barrier between us, chatting with the nurses about his kids and their acting-out proclivities, his great head of hair inches from my face the whole time. Only local anesthesia was required, and given the lack of sensation in my chest, even that was hardly necessary.

But within a few days, my left side, dressed only with my original thin, sensitive breast skin, reacted to the adhesive that held the bandages in place. The skin blistered and peeled, taking the entire surgically constructed nipple with it. My right side, armored with tougher skin harvested from my back, fared better, and after a few weeks, I had a surprisingly natural-looking button of a nipple on the right, just where it should be.

So we tried again, a few months later, with the left side. This time, Dr. Smith used no adhesives and used special non-reactive antiseptics, just in case, and in time, the left side perfectly matched the right. Of course. Because Dr. Smith is the perfectionist you want your plastic surgeon to be. A few months later, I spent an hour in Dr. Smith's office with the tattoo artist, who was kind and compassionate, and drew out my entire story during our time together, even though she'd heard hundreds of similar stories before.

And suddenly, just like that, I was done. As complete a woman as I was ever again going to be, at least physically. I didn't even bother with the follow-up call a week later to them know how I was doing. I was doing fine.

•   •   •   •   •

Reconstruction preserves the form, the aesthetic, of a female body, but not the function. Reconstructed breasts are muscle and skin, stretched over silicon balloons, then stitched in place. The nerves, even to the skin, are offline. The only sensation I have now is a constant, low-grade itching, for which scratching is no relief, like the pain in a phantom limb, and a banded tightness around my chest.

In 2010, I didn't know if preserving that aesthetic would be important to me, or to Jeff, with whom I have shared this body for 35 years. At the time, it felt like a big risk to come out of the mastectomy with a completely flat terrain. What if I was horrified? What if he was? I thought that preserving form, even without function, would at least cushion the impact of this crisis.

Since 2010, I have thought a lot about whether all of this—from the Growing Up Skipper expansion to the areola tattoos—was worth it. Of course, the mastectomy—saving my life—was worth it. But the reconstruction was optional. Did it, in fact, soften the crisis? Would I do it again?

As I write this, I've just turned 54. I can start to see 60 up ahead, and I contemplate whether I will still care about having breasts when I'm 60. Breast implants need to be re-done every ten years. So as I edge towards 60, I will stumble over my ten-year cancer anniversary and must decide what to do next. *Now* how important is this female form I carry through the world? Then again at 70—how about *now*? Then 80—how about *now*? (At 80, surely not, I think. But what do I know?)

Even six years into my time inhabiting this transformed body, it feels like a different question than in 2010. It's tomato versus tomaato and potato versus potaato. I'm not the same person now. I don't have the same body, cancer completely aside. Truthfully, at 54, I don't seem to care that much about having breasts. I also no longer care that much about being a few pounds overweight or being seen in a crappy t-shirt at the grocery. I've moved into a different stage of life, with different priorities and a different set of expectations about what it means to be female. Jeff and I are both older. It's not that the ardor has cooled, but the river of hormones has definitely slowed. Often, the wisdom from Yenta, the matchmaker, in Fiddler on the Roof, bounces through my head: With the way he sees and the way she looks, it's a perfect match!

And yet, reconstruction allowed me a few years to come to terms with the fact that my breasts are gone. Although reconstruction may be a purely aesthetic choice, the aesthetic mattered in my recovery from cancer. For six years, having reconstructed "breasts" has allowed me to feel more or less normal when I get up in the morning and go to bed at night, despite the un-scratchable itching and the feeling that I'm perpetually bound by an Ace bandage. I don't have to stuff a bra with prostheses every day. I can wear a t-shirt without a bra in the summer, and probably no one notices. I can change my clothes in a locker room without feeling like a freak show. There's a lot to be said for a return to normal, or a simulated normal, and for moving through the world unencumbered by physical reminders of grief. Normal allowed me to shift away from cancer as much as I could.

But the importance of that aesthetic has dimmed over time. I've gotten used to this new body, the body that has allowed me to navigate the world in a simulated normal. I realize now that I could probably get used to a different normal — whatever I decide that will be.

This is the good news about breast reconstruction. You can change your mind. The decision is both flexible and revocable. When I made the decision in 2010, Dr. Smith emphasized that I could choose not to have reconstruction with the mastectomy, but still choose it later. In fact, reconstruction is an option at any point after mastectomy, and insurance still must pay. I chose to go ahead at mastectomy time, to avoid multiple surgeries (so much for that plan). But I could have waited. Now I can make a different choice.

So now, several years in front of the next decision point, I daydream about the amazing tattoo I could have on the flat terrain of my chest, reconstruction left behind. A tree of life, branches unfurling from my sternum, a trunk following the contours of my ribcage, and roots vining towards my navel. A dragon, breathing fire across my heart, its tail curving around my right side and catching the reconstruction surgery scar on my back. A thicket of red roses, a tangle of thorns and blossoms, the substance of a rich and complicated life. The possibilities are endless.

I joke that I'm going to get the tattoo for my sixtieth birthday, that I'm starting to save my pennies now. But maybe sixty is too far away. Maybe the tattoo is right around the corner, waiting to transform my body once again into something new and mysterious. A body that, with luck, will carry me into the ethereal final three decades of my life.

•   •   •   •   •

In 2013, about a month after I fell on the water-slick kitchen floor of our Minneapolis apartment, I fell again. We were walking home to the apartment on an icy winter night after an easy evening of jazz and martinis. We'd just walked past the Cancer Survivors Park a few blocks from home, which I had taken to calling the Fuck Cancer Park.

The ice struck, once again. Despite my practical winter boots, despite my mostly sober state. Swoosh, down. The ice-misted, grey night sky, tinged with the cinnamon streetlights of Minneapolis, wet and cold as a dog's nose, gazed impassively down at me as the frozen concrete pressed up from below.

I lay there and thought: I can believe this is strike two, game two, and that strike three looms around the pointy corner of next month. Or I can believe that I am kind of a klutz, and I really should hang onto Jeff's arm more firmly in icy conditions. Which is it?

Jeff helped me up, and we continued towards home, arm in arm.

A few weeks later, I found a lump in my upper left arm about the size of a large marble—a shooter, as we used to call them—or a fat green grape ready to burst on the tongue. My heart stopped beating for a moment, then chugged in at twice its previous speed. I called the oncologist the next day, and commenced the now familiar round of exam, ultrasound, biopsy, waiting, phone call. I had been around this track several times now, post-cancer, because when you've had as much cancer as I'd had, the checkered flags drop as soon as the smallest lump appears.

The news was good. Just some scar tissue, appearing out of nowhere. No explanation. Let us know if it gets bigger or causes you discomfort.

Maybe my in-utero twin, I thought. Migrated to the underside of my left upper arm. Which made about as much sense as anything else in the past three years. You do hear about such things, after all.

I breathed another sigh of relief and turned my sights back to the road ahead.

•   •   •   •   •

When we moved back to our house that summer, leaving behind the Stone Arch Bridge and the Mississippi River, I decided it was time. Although I'd known in the quiet of Sam's hospital room that I needed to let go, it had taken me a while to get there.

I got a box from the garage, then went through all of the cupboards and closets and drawers in the house, rooting out the detritus I'd kept for three years, the fetid talismen against cancer. I took the ginger ale and unopened ginger thins and ginger candy to the food shelf. I threw out the KY Jelly and the constipation remedies and the half-full bottles of supplements. I donated the hats and scarves and cut the cancer pants up into cleaning rags. I took the pain medication and anti-anxiety drugs and muscle relaxants to the police station safe disposal box, and put the sample-sized tubes of Aquaphor into all my purses and rechristened it as lip balm.

I knew all along that I'd been keeping a double set of books. The magical: falling down three times meant I'd struck out, which set me up for cancer; and keeping the debris of cancer around would keep me safe from round two. The rational: things don't Happen for a Reason. It's an impersonal universe.

If I let go of the magical thinking, it meant I had to let go of the idea that adversity was predictable or within my control. But it didn't necessarily mean that life's satisfactions were not within my control. In fact, deciding that life is good, despite the adversity, had been within my control all along. Maybe cancer didn't happen to teach me lessons. But I could learn them anyway.

It had taken me a few years to get here. But I no longer needed that magical thinking. I was ready to give it up, or at least fence it in, where even if I could not eliminate it entirely, I could at least keep an eye on it.

There's always more ginger ale in the world, I thought, and doctors ready to write pain med scripts. There are endless bowls of Aquaphor samples, free for the taking, and less scruffy cancer pants, and caring people to knit me more hats. I decided to give up my fear of uncertainty and move into the world of exhilarating unknowns, where I would be okay, no matter what.

•   •   •   •   •

In the spring of 2014, Jeff and I picked up four more state parks by visiting the southwest corner of the state on a warm spring weekend. The weekend before had been unseasonably cold, and an ice storm had caused iced-over birds to literally fall from the sky, unable to sustain their northward migration another hour, past the calamity of the storm. Talk about Stupid Metaphors. I could identify.

Blue Mounds State Park features a swath of original prairie, complete with roaming buffalo. I think some deer and antelope still play there, even. In some distant geologic era, the prairie split open to reveal thirty- to forty-foot high cliffs of pink quartzite, now popular with rock climbers and cliff swallows.

I could not ignore the fact that these cliffs were pink. Pink had become something other than just a color I didn't much care for. It felt ominous and threatening, at least metaphorically. As I clambered over the pink boulders, I stopped to gaze out across the still-brown prairie that stretched into the distance. The April sun shone down, and I'd tied my sweatshirt around my waist to cool off. But when my hand explored the crevices between the boulders, the air was icy cold.

I'd taken those two falls last year, one in our apartment, one on the icy street. So I must be due for strike three. Wouldn't it be just great to take my final fall here, I thought, from the pink cliff to the hard ground in a matter of seconds? Wouldn't that just sum it all up? What a great ending to my story.

That's what cancer will do to your head.

Jeff clambered past me, then turned and reached out his hand. I clutched it firmly, finding my footing as he helped haul me up and over the rocks. Which were, after all, just rocks.

Chapter Twenty-Two

It's August 2016, and it's corn season. Every night, I put the pot on to boil, then shuck the corn, inhaling the fresh, green scent—essence of corn. My hands get a little sticky from the kernel milk that leaks when I dig too deep or snap an inch of stalk off the end of the cob. As I pull away stray strands of silk, I think: I made it another year.

I count my years by corn seasons now. This is my sixth year since cancer. I am six years old, in corn-seasons.

In August of 2010, as I navigated doctors and procedures by day and boiled the corn at night, I was keenly aware that real corn-on-the-cob—straight from the Minnesota field—only happens once a year, for about a month. Sure, you can get corn in the frozen foods section or as a side at the barbeque joint. But it's not worth eating.

Throughout that cancer year, and the next several years, the question worried me. Would I live to see another corn season?

We will all get there eventually. The time when we will never again eat fresh corn, or Washington sweet cherries (another limited season favorite), or our mother's chocolate cake, or a steak seared to perfection. There will be a final great martini, a last time we embrace a beloved child or look into a lover's eyes. We may or may not know it when it happens, but it will happen.

My diagnosis was not terminal, so I don't yet know what it's like to live with that reality—knowing each singular experience may be the last. And the good news is, these years later I have stopped thinking in these terms. Now I don't automatically think, this may be my last birthday or my last Thanksgiving or my last trip to Chicago. I have regained my footing in the world, my near certainty that life will go on for a good long time, so I can sit back and let it happen. Sure, I could get hit by a truck anytime. But it seems pretty unlikely.

So maybe, from this vantage point, corn season marks my rebirth, my re-emergence into life, on the other side of trauma. It's a lovely, long month when the garden is lush, the weather is fine, and we all take a good, deep breath before the busy-ness of fall descends. It's a time to enjoy what's in season, knowing that although it will come around again, the time to indulge is now.

·   ·   ·   ·   ·

Recently, I was on my way to my yearly oncology appointment, six years out from my initial diagnosis. As I drove between the green fields lining the corn corridor, I noticed they were mostly planted in soybeans this year.

Huh, I thought. Things change.

For so long, I didn't want to be changed by cancer. But, of course, cancer changed me.

I know that a lot of people who experience cancer come away feeling like it somehow righted their course. Their inner fiber was proofed in the fire and emerged with a new strength. Pig iron to steel. I once was lost, but now am found. They find God, or reunite with their estranged family, or quit the hated job and move to Belize to live on the beach. That's supposed to be the bright side of cancer. You Wake Up and Smell the Coffee.

But when I was diagnosed with cancer, I believed I could already smell the coffee. I was stopping along every freaking path, to smell every cup, and every rose besides. I loved my life. I had a great family, great kids, and a whole bunch of great friends. I liked my work. God and I, we had come to terms, as had Jeff and I. It wasn't that I didn't have problems and anxieties and complaints. But I believed that I did not want to change a single thing that was within my power to change. And I was not wrong.

But I wonder now if I resisted the idea that cancer would change me because I wanted to have lived my life well, with no regrets, all along. That I didn't need anything to change. At an early age, I'd decided I needed to do this on my own. And in doing it on my own, I wanted to be blameless, as if I had something to prove. See? I can do this without help, and I can do it right, besides. I made choices, and they were good choices that led to a reasonably happy life. I didn't need cancer to teach me lessons, like a fusty old school teacher insisting on his way. I didn't need help from anywhere.

Now I see cancer as a dynamic in my life, rather than an obstacle to overcome as quickly as possible and then move beyond, forgotten on the road. A dynamic can come and go, take on different dimensions at different times, and foster growth. But seeing cancer, and other life surprises, as dynamics rather than as obstacles required me to shift. I had to see that I could possibly take a wrong turn. I had maybe even done so. But it would be okay even if I had. I would find my way again.

I think here is where the threads weave together. The warp and the woof of freedom and responsibility are fundamental. But there's another ingredient in the weave: mystery. There is so much mystery in why things happen to us and why we can't control them, no matter how hard we try. With cancer, I have come to accept that I will never answer the questions that provoked me for so long: why me? Did I bring this on myself? What should I have done differently?

Maybe I *was* to blame, because of my microwaved lunches or my unresolved issues or my cloud of bug spray. Maybe I could have done something differently. Maybe not. Maybe blame is beside the point. Sometimes what happens to us is a mystery. But we can take credit for how we respond.

As I navigated the terrain in the cancerland jungle, I learned that I was up to it. I could keep picking myself up and moving on, with a little help from my family, my friends, and some total strangers. I learned that accepting help did not make me weak or more vulnerable. And that despite the need to pick myself up over and over again, I was happy. Life was still worth living. I wanted more, please.

I have to admit: those seem like important lessons.

· · · · ·

You want to know what lessons cancer taught me? Here's The Big One: Life is too short to finish *War and Peace*.

My hyper-intellectual couples reading group, in which, among us, we have a total of several dozen advanced degrees, had been talking about reading *War and Peace* for years. We finally decided to go for it last winter.

I was game. I like a challenge. I like goals. I almost never abandon a book in the middle. I believe that reading Big Books builds character.

But a few hundred pages in, a thought kept poking me, distracting me from the carnage among the Russian troops. The thought was this: in my new, post-cancer status, I was counting the moments in a more intentional way than I ever had before. And I was unwilling to devote any of my remaining moments to an activity as boring as this. I put the book down.

Since then, I've had the same reaction to dental hygiene lectures, but more overtly hostile. If my mouth were not full of bony, latex-covered hands and cold metal during the lecture, I would spit the words out with a side of venom: I'm too old and have been through too much to sit through one more earnest explanation of the perils of unflossed dentalia. Stop wasting my time. I don't have that much, in total.

Next time, I'm going to bite someone.

Other "life's too short" issues require some thought, some balance, less viscera in the decision sandwich. I contemplate the second (or third) cookie, the warm chocolate lava cake on the dessert menu, the second Dragon Margarita, and I think: which principle wins here? Live life to the fullest in every moment? Or live healthily over the long term, including keeping the weight under control, to optimize longevity? Clearly, I can't always choose both.

Nowadays, these decisions, and the decisions about what nonsense to put up with from moment to moment, wind themselves back to cancer and what it means to have endured it. I know that if I actually *had* terminal cancer, I would eat the cookie and order another margarita. I decided that a couple of years ago. But I don't actually *have* terminal cancer, and I do want to live a long time, and at a reasonable weight, and in reasonably good health. So my contention that metaphorically we all have cancer, of a sort—because we're all going to die—and should live accordingly, doesn't stand up to practical scrutiny. We can't be simultaneously farsighted, our eyes focused sharply on the distant horizon, and nearsighted, our eyes narrowed on the still life in front of us. We have to live somewhere in the middle, finding our bliss well enough every day, but mindful that we need to have the stamina to get to the end.

So now, when I'm faced with some irritating but mundane task, like getting that last bit of expensive moisturizer out of the tube or searching for airline tickets just a little bit cheaper, I think: if I had stage IV cancer, I would not do this. Then I allow myself to not do it anyway, because this moment isn't any less valuable just because my death is probably years away rather than months away.

Thus, once again, I can't plausibly say my life was not changed by cancer, although that's what I wanted to claim for so long. I've been an unreliable narrator in that respect, my confirmation bias chugging away like everyone else's. My life *was* irrevocably changed by cancer. But it is also changed just by getting out of bed every morning and tackling whatever comes down the pike. I have to remember to take that opportunity for change into account, alongside everything on my gratitude list.

• • • • •

Let's return to the Fuck Cancer Park for a moment. As I hope I've made clear, I don't believe I'm a hero because I've survived cancer. Everyone must experience the debacle of cancer in their own way, and some cancer sufferers truly are heroic: children with cancer, for instance, and those whose cancer experience is more devastating and painful than mine. People who are certain to die of cancer, but live for years in beautiful and meaningful ways. But for me, cancer just happened, and I dealt with it because I didn't want to die yet. I would have done the same if my house had fallen into a sinkhole, or an asteroid had crashed into my yard, or a prehistoric monster had risen from the Cannon River and chased me down Division Street. I would have climbed out, or run as fast as I could, or taken whatever other action the situation required. And I believe that other than getting out of the way, so the beast does not devour you, your reaction should be to shake your tiny fist at the sky and shout: I'm not ready yet, so fuck you! Go away! And don't come back until I'm good and ready!

That's not to say that people who experience cancer are not courageous and admirable and deserving of all the help we can give them. Of course they are. But really, what have I survived that can't be lumped in with all the other tragedies of the human condition? Shit happens, and some shit stinks more than other shit, and we should do our best to hold our noses and move on. And by "do our best," I mean, continue to live as richly and fully as possible, with joy and gratitude, no matter what troubles befall us, even though that is sometimes extremely difficult to pull off. The inventory that made my life meaningful during cancer parallels the inventory that made my life meaningful before and after cancer: the comfort of family, a meal and conversation with friends, satisfying work, music in my ears at all hours, good books, long hikes in state parks, dark chocolate, white cupcakes, fresh organic greens, dog walks on frigid mornings, Minnesota corn-on-the-cob, eagles soaring over the Mississippi River, a martini shaken by the hands of my sweetheart, served in a chilled glass, and sipped with friends. None of that changed. I didn't survive cancer. I endured the inconvenience of cancer, with as much grace as I could muster, while living my life as best I could.

But I recognize that I went through a lot and it took something to get through it. And sometimes people ask me: what did it take?

When I consider that question—how did I work my way through the interminable downs and ups and cutting and stitching and barfing and discomfort and grief that came with cancer—I usually shrug and say, it's just what anyone would do.

But recently, I stumbled onto the literature about why certain children thrive, even when presented with difficult circumstances. After some reading, I put a sticky note on my bulletin board listing qualities that the experts say feed "character": zest, grit, self-control, social intelligence, gratitude, optimism, and curiosity.

I am squeamish about applying these ideas to myself. I'll leave it to others to decide how I measure up. But the ideas resonate, at least as qualities I aspire to. To thrive through adversity, I believe you have to continue to love your life, despite the moments when you want to die. You have to keep hiking up that bluff and resist the urge to turn around or jump. You have to cherish your social network and pay it forward, both before and after your own crisis. You have to recognize the gifts that the world bestows on you in the form of love, support, and material comforts, and appreciate them every day. You have to envision the next thirty years and be all-in to see what happens down that road. You have to believe you will beat this, whatever the challenge is.

Fostering these qualities might not mean you will live forever. But it means you will continue to live for now.

So please, when I die, whether it's next year, as I sometimes dream about—my death announcement crowded on the lower corner of the Northfield News front page—or years from now, at age 103, don't say I died "after a heroic battle with cancer," as so many obituaries do. Every moment of life is fraught with challenging, exhilarating, terrifying peril. And we don't survive it. We live it, and then we die. The trick is not to survive. It's to live the whole time.

Epilogue

On a warm September afternoon, Ruby lay out in the yard whimpering, barely able to move. In the previous week, the vet had x-rayed her bones and, with the help of light anesthesia, thoroughly prodded her soft tissue. We had tried several pain medications, all to no avail. The diagnosis wasn't clear, but she was in extreme pain and couldn't walk. Maybe serious disk disease. Maybe a tumor on the spine that did not appear on the x-ray.

I couldn't eat my dinner, and I couldn't work or read. Jeff went out for the evening, and I sat in the kitchen feeling helpless and grief-stricken. I was convinced that the next day, after a night of suffering, Ruby's back end would be paralyzed, and she would be unable to rise from the ground or tend to her bodily functions. The vet would have to make a house call to bring her life to an artificial end. She weighed 106 pounds, and we couldn't get her in the car.

I called my sister Ann to talk through my grief. As I sobbed into the phone, she said, just go out and sit with her. Pet her ears, stroke her fur. You know what she likes. You'll both feel better, even if you can't ease her pain.

So I stuffed my wad of tissues into my pocket, then retrieved the orange nylon sleeping bag, untouched in the garage since the state park trip in 2010, the week before my cancer diagnosis. I went in the yard and spread the sleeping bag on the sweet-smelling, leaf-covered ground next to her. I made my way down to the ground and pulled myself close to her. I ran my hand down the long, luxurious fur that cloaks her shoulders, and dug my fingers deep into the shorter fur that carpets the folds around her neck, where she likes to be scratched. I stroked her ears and her front paws and ran my thumb down the black bandit mask between her eyes. When I stopped moving my hand, she feebly raised a paw to remind me to keep going.

I lay on the ground next to her for about an hour, petting her and crying. There was nothing else I could do for this companion on my life's journey. The September night air was warm, and since there'd been no rain for a week, the earth under my sleeping bag was dry and comfortable.

I remembered letting her off the leash at the county wilderness park when she was young and at her athletic peak. She could run for hours without stopping, around and around us in huge circuits as we hiked. Splashing down the creek, splashing up the creek. Down the hill, up the hill, then back down the hill and back up the hill, stopping briefly at the top to grin at us, tongue lolling, before taking off again, as if she had to be in Nome with the vaccine by noon. Even in the confines of the yard, she would run in endless joyful circles, or in crazy trajectories to fetch the ball, stopping just short of the fence, where she could execute a hairpin turn just in the nick of time. She would dig a hole deep enough to bury a pony and emerge covered in mud, wagging from snout to tail. If she escaped the house without a leash, it took forever to corral her. She was a genius at getting just close enough to give you hope as you lunged for her collar, then taking off for another pass around the neighborhood, until you were ready to cry with frustration and fatigue.

I could do nothing to ease her suffering that night, other than lie next to her, stroking her fur. Telling her what a good dog she was and that everything would be okay. I put my tear-runny nose next to hers, and I looked up at the clear September sky, where the stars twinkled down at us through the locust trees. She closed her eyes and sighed.

Taking care of each other, being present through the suffering, is not a new game. It's the oldest game of all.

NOTE FROM THE AUTHOR

Word-of-mouth is crucial for any author to succeed. If you enjoyed the book, please leave a review online—anywhere you are able. Even if it's just a sentence or two. It would make all the difference and would be very much appreciated.

Thanks!
Mary

About the Author

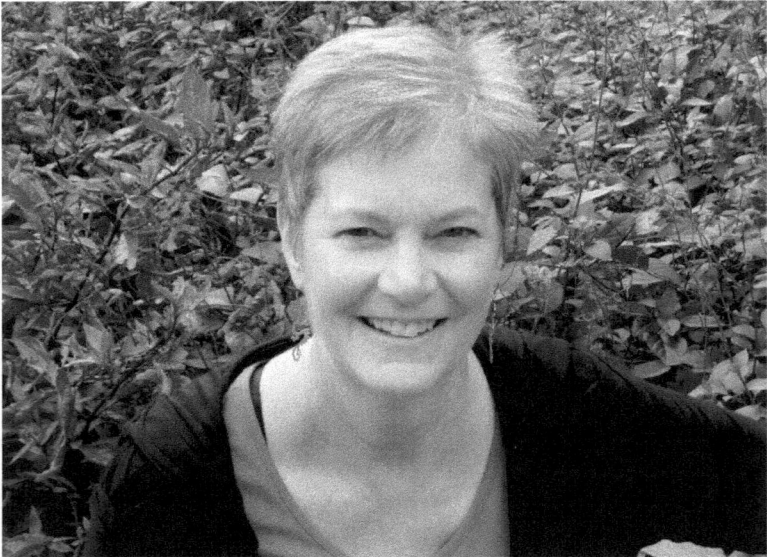

Mary Dunnewold is a writer, lawyer, and educator. She holds a BA from St. Olaf College, an MA from the University of Minnesota, and a JD from the University of Minnesota School of Law. She lives in Northfield, Minnesota, where the sign welcoming visitors to town promises, "Cows, Colleges, and Contentment." Mostly, the town follows through on that promise.

Thank you so much for reading one of our **Biography / Memoirs**.

If you enjoyed our book, please check out our recommended title for your next great read!

Z.O.S. by Kay Merkel Boruff

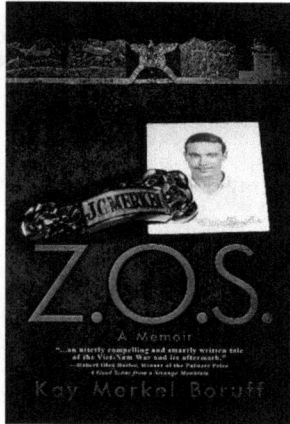

"...dazzling in its specificity and intensity."

–C.W. Smith, author of *Understanding Women*

www.ingramcontent.com/pod-product-compliance
Lightning Source LLC
Chambersburg PA
CBHW060318030426
42336CB00011B/1112